More praise for *Talking to Depression*

"This book recognizes the power of altruism in healing, and the capacities of a depressed person to herself be a healer for others . . . Strauss not only suggests how we can be a good friend to a friend who is depressed, but she provides us instructions on *how* to be a good friend. [*Talking to Depression* is] a really important tool for knowing how to relate and how to connect when people in your life are struggling with depression."

—Jo Cohen Hamilton, PhD, professor of counseling
and human services at Kutztown University

"*Talking to Depression* is a war chest of tools to aid our understanding of something that defies understanding unless one has experienced it first-hand . . . In an ideal world [this book] would not be needed. The next best thing would be that it finds its way into every home and library. Perhaps, in the right hands, this book could save lives."

—Christine B. Smith, PhD, president of S.O.L.O.S., Inc.
(Survivors of Loved Ones' Suicide)

"Ms. Strauss has created a wonderfully helpful book for all of us. An excellent manual for the day to day interaction with the depressed person. This book would be a wonderful addition to anyone's library that unfortunately will get excellent use!"   —Peter A. Schwartz, M.D.

"It is an essential read for the layperson that does not understand the experience of depression and wants to help a friend or family member through it . . . practical ideas, common sense guidelines and clear explanations that can make a difference in the lives of those with depression."

—Marta C. Peck, executive director of the Mental
Health Association of Reading & Berks County

continued . . .

"This book is about what the person suffering from depression needs to hear and, even more importantly, about what that person should *not* hear . . . Strauss doesn't just give the persons with depression a chance to get the daily support they need, she gives the people who love them a way to feel renewed in their own lives. I found it enlightening, inspiring, and enormously instructive."

—Nancy Wolter Brooks, speech pathologist, and health, rehabilitation, and social work professional

"I can't say enough about Claudia Strauss's manuscript, *Talking to Depression*. This is definitely a guide that is needed. I've never seen anything that addresses friends and family in this way—and so thoroughly, so compassionately, yet so simply. What a contribution to the field!"

—Michelle L. Hostetter, Psy.D., clinical psychologist

Talking
to
Eating Disorders

Simple Ways to
Support Someone with
Anorexia, Bulimia, Binge Eating,
or Body Image Issues

JEANNE ALBRONDA HEATON, PH.D.
AND CLAUDIA J. STRAUSS

New American Library

New American Library
Published by New American Library, a division of
Penguin Group (USA) Inc., 375 Hudson Street,
New York, New York 10014, USA
Penguin Group (Canada), 90 Eglinton Avenue, Suite 700, Toronto,
Ontario M4P 2Y3 Canada (a division of Pearson Penguin Canada Inc.)
Penguin Books Ltd., 80 Strand, London WC2R 0RL, England
Penguin Ireland, 25 St. Stephen's Green, Dublin 2,
Ireland (a division of Penguin Books Ltd.)
Penguin Group (Australia), 250 Camberwell Road, Camberwell, Victoria 3124,
Australia (a division of Pearson Australia Group Pty. Ltd.)
Penguin Books India Pvt. Ltd., 11 Community Centre, Panchsheel Park,
New Delhi - 110 017, India
Penguin Group (NZ), cnr Airborne and Rosedale Roads, Albany,
Auckland 1310, New Zealand (a division of Pearson New Zealand Ltd.)
Penguin Books (South Africa) (Pty.) Ltd., 24 Sturdee Avenue,
Rosebank, Johannesburg 2196, South Africa

Penguin Books Ltd., Registered Offices:
80 Strand, London WC2R 0RL, England

First published by New American Library,
a division of Penguin Group (USA) Inc.

First Printing, July 2005
10 9 8 7 6 5 4

NEW AMERICAN LIBRARY and logo are trademarks of Penguin Group (USA) Inc.

LIBRARY OF CONGRESS CATALOGING-IN-PUBLICATION DATA:

Heaton, Jeanne Albronda, 1944–
Talking to eating disorders : simple ways to support someone who has anorexia, bulimia binge eating,
or body image issues / by Jeanne Albronda Heaton, Claudia J. Strauss.
p. cm.
Includes bibliographical references.
ISBN 0-451-21522-2
1. Eating disorders—Patients—Family relationships. 2. Eating disorders—Patients—
Counseling of. I. Strauss, Claudia, J., 1952–   II. Title.
RC522.E18H43 2005
362.2'5—dc22   2005006150

Printed in the United States of America

PUBLISHER'S NOTE
While the author has made every effort to provide accurate telephone numbers and Internet addresses at
the time of publication, neither the publisher nor the author assumes any responsibility for errors, or for
changes that occur after publication. Further, publisher does not have any control over and does not assume any responsibility for author or third-party Web sites or their content.

Acknowledgments

I would like to thank my clients. You have taught me most of what I know about helping people. Your willingness to trust me with your secrets, to confront me when I was off base, and to try again when that seemed impossible inspires me to share what I've learned from you about eating problems. And I'd like to acknowledge the people who read this book who will do so because they care enough to help others who endure these isolating and punishing problems. Your efforts can help those who live day to day with eating disorders to feel better, do better, and suffer much less.

Next, I would like to thank Charlotte Kasl, a lifelong friend, who put me in touch with Edite Kroll, my agent, who cared enough to talk me through all the initial stages of writing this book, and who put me in touch with Tracy Bernstein, the editor at NAL who had the wisdom to see that working with Claudia Strauss would be the great idea it has turned out to be. I'm grateful to have the opportunity to work with such talented professionals who care not only about what they are doing but about the people they are doing it with. I would like to thank Shannon O'Leary and Karen Williams for their thoughtful editorial comments. I dedicate this to my family because I treasure their friendship, and to my friends who make me feel like family.

I dedicate this to my family because I treasure their friendship, and to my friends who make me feel like family.

—Jeanne Albronda Heaton, Ph.D.

v

* * *

I would like to thank all the people who contributed to my knowledge on this subject and all those who carefully read what I had written. They drew on their own experience with various forms of eating disorders, variously as people suffering, in recovery, and with fully restored and rewarding lives; as people who counsel others facing the same devastating challenges; and as parents and friends who struggled and watched and experimented and learned. And I would like to thank those who awakened me to the power of these disorders and the way they take over people's lives. Friends and students over the years have long made me want to find a way to help. You have all played a vital role in ensuring not only the effectiveness of what is suggested here but also the way the words themselves will be received. I wish I could list all of you here: Dana Wurtz, Andrea Bloomgarden, Nikita Samborski, Maura Buzad, Jim Ingrund, Deidre Brown, Amy Squibb, Michelle Hostetter, Joan Hastings, Lane Aikens, Jane Fleming, Marta Peck, Andrea Dillaway-Huber, Leigh Cohn, Stephanie Muller, Roberto Olivardia, Pat Wilson, Beth Wells, Sister Sharon Susin, Ann Klein, Deborah Wurtz.

I am grateful to Claire Zion and Tracy Bernstein for involving me in this project, and to Jeanne Heaton for welcoming my participation. I hope that this book will help many caring people help their friends, family members, students, and coworkers navigate these difficult waters and not feel quite so overwhelmed.

I dedicate this book to all the people I hope it can help, whether you are struggling with an eating disorder yourself or whether you are trying to be there for someone who is. It is a hard road; I hope this book can help you walk it together.

—Claudia J. Strauss

Contents

Contents

PART III SPECIAL ISSUES: GOING THE DISTANCE

At least do no harm.

∞—HIPPOCRATES

Introduction

∽

$\mathcal{F}$or each one of the millions of people afflicted with an eating problem, there are many others significantly affected by their problems—people like you. Whether you're a family member, teacher, religious adviser, coach, friend, or coworker, you need to know that *you can make a difference.*

It's baffling to watch someone struggle with a problem that "makes no sense." Of course it's ridiculous to eat thousands of calories, only to throw them up. Everyone knows it's a bad idea not to eat at all for a week. And most assuredly, it is frightening to watch someone continue to binge on chocolate after being told by a doctor "your blood pressure is too high and your diabetes is out of control."

The pursuit of a better life through a better body has led millions into the turmoil of yo-yo dieting and the accompanying self-contempt that underlies most eating problems. To add to the problem, the actors and models we see in magazines, on television, and in the movies are significantly thinner and often more muscular than the people we see around us. (What we don't see are the health risks these people have taken: e.g., amenorrhea, osteoporotic bones, surgery to eliminate ribs, legal or illegal drugs to keep going and reduce appetite.) These masterfully constructed images, which are usually computer-enhanced, beckon us to pursue the fantasy that we too can be "better," "thinner"—"more perfect." As a nation, we've bought into a preoccupation with weight that has millions dieting and exercising and an unfortunate number sinking into the mental torture associated with anorexia, bulimia, and binge eating.

Because each of us affected by the craziness that encircles these eating problems is also influenced by the same culture that contributed to the development of these problems in the first place, it's not surprising that most people are confused about how to help.

Friends and family usually begin by applauding the efforts of their loved one to lose weight and come closer to "that perfect image." But when those diets backfire into compulsive overeating, binge eating, bulimia or anorexia, we former supporters move from approval to concern. We've all been warned by the surgeon general that obesity kills, and we've heard about people like Karen Carpenter who died of bulimia and anorexia.

We are alarmed when we notice the problem, and feel guilty if we don't do something about it. We also worry about damaging our relationships with our efforts to help. It is difficult to stay in our role as friend, family member, or coworker because people with eating disorders are often artful dodgers; one minute they seem open to what we have to say and the next minute they are apt to be insulting and rude, or worse, may close us out altogether.

Because we care about the suffering we observe, we want to fix these problem quickly. Usually that leads us to push for solutions, such as to start exercising, eat more, eat less, or stop vomiting. But if suggesting these obvious solutions were all that curing an eating disorder required, no one would be ill! The first thing to realize is that you can't simply order up change, even desired change.

However, you can still help. This book will help you figure out how.

Even if you have had these problems yourself, you can help. Even more important, you don't have to have all your difficulties solved before you can help another person with eating disorders. In fact, as Gloria Steinem wisely said, "We often teach what we need to learn." (1.) A special word to those of you who are dieticians, counselors, or doctors who have friends and family suffering from eating disorders: You already know that you need to follow the ethical guidelines of your profession by not treating your family members or friends, but you'll also want to avoid falling into the trap of reacting to them as though your relationship were a professional one.

DIFFERENT TERMS—SIMILAR ISSUES

The problems we are going to discuss are:

- **Anorexia:** The inability to maintain normal weight for age and height. While there is no exact cut-off, many consider going below 85 percent of expected weight range while still fearing being fat or "not being thin enough" is an indication of anorexia. People with anorexia lose weight either by restricting what they eat (anorexia/restricting type) or by bingeing and purging (anorexia—binge eating/purging type).
- **Bulimia:** Characterized by periods of bingeing (although sometimes it's just normal amounts of food) followed by self-induced vomiting, intake of laxatives or diuretics, obsessive exercise and/or periods of starvation.
- **Binge-eating disorder** (BED): Periodically eating large amounts of food or compulsive periods of excessive eating.

These may seem like different problems, but they are all tied together. When people try to manage weight while also trying to satisfy basic biological needs for fuel they begin a treacherous journey on a very tight rope. A few manage okay and reach the other side—satisfied with their ability to balance. However, many teeter between the restricting (dieting) side and the indulgence (bingeing) side. Some people sway back and forth so wildly that they fall (meaning they get an eating disorder). Eating disorders represent a loss of balance, because what people with eating disorders are trying to do isn't based on what their bodies need. Quite simply, they are trying to force unworkable solutions on demanding bodies.

Tired and stressed, the people we are concerned about will swing between effort and avoidance. Acutely aware of failure, many redouble their efforts. Most feel ashamed of their behavior and guilty because they recognize that what they are doing isn't healthy. Eventually, their moods are controlled by their weight loss efforts and failures. Their mood is up with weight loss and down with weight gain—nothing else matters as much. In addition, people who don't eat properly tend to be cranky, irritable, anxious, worried, and preoccupied. They're secretive. Most important, they're often hard to relate to.

You don't need to analyze or even understand the psychological underpinnings of eating disorders to be an effective helper. You will gain more peace of mind from figuring out what you *can* do rather than trying to figure out what's wrong and what caused this eating disorder to develop in the first place. Consider the Zen proverb: "If you understand, things are just as they are; if you do not understand, things are just as they are." Most important, whatever your role—whether that is to be a parent, a partner, a sister, a teacher, a coach, a friend—your relationship can serve as an essential foundation for improvement.

Therapy can be very helpful when a person is ready, and we'll help you figure out how to motivate someone to seek professional help. But many if not most people with eating problems never see a therapist at all. And even if the person you're worried about is getting professional help, there are many more hours of the day when she'll need the support and encouragement of those who care.

We have teamed up to write this book because we believe the information from both a psychologist experienced in working with eating disorders and an author of several books on how to talk about difficult topics will give you the benefit of what we both have learned about helping others without making the problem worse. This material is organized to help you help the person or people you are worried about.

HOW TO USE THIS BOOK

In the first section of this book, you will learn why blaming yourself—or anyone else, for that matter—won't help. You'll learn how to encourage change, with specific suggestions for how to talk to people who are at different stages of changing. For example, some people haven't admitted to a problem at all, whereas others will have already made some significant gains. We'll help you figure out how to manage the withdrawal, tears, anger, and lying that accompany many eating problems, and how to make your conversations more effective.

The third section will help you tackle tough topics that inevitably accompany most eating problems: body-image concerns, messages from the media, food choices and dieting, exercise regimens, getting professional help, managing emergencies, and staying the course once the person you care about is better. There is also a special chapter for talking to kids about their own and other people's eating problems.

AN EDITORIAL NOTE

We think readers will get the most out of this book if they read it from start to finish, but if you happen to be in the middle of a crisis, we suggest that you read the first four chapters and then skip to chapter twelve on managing emergencies.

In this book we will usually use the term "we" to refer to all of us who know someone struggling with an eating disorder. Occasionally, as in this paragraph, we use the term "we" to mean the authors; the meaning should be clear from the context.

We know that eating disorders are hard for both men and women, so we have used "he" and "she" interchangeably.

This book was written to help you know what to say to people you care about. Many of the suggestions offered here will be useful for those who might not have a full-fledged eating disorder. It's never too early to express the concern you feel. Most relationships benefit from an open expression of thoughts, feelings, and concerns.

Part I

∞

ENCOURAGING CHANGE:
WHAT IT TAKES

A mistake is evidence that somebody has tried to accomplish something.

Chapter One

Replacing Blame with Respect

∞

*T*hink for a moment about the person you want to talk to when you need support, advice, and understanding. That person makes you feel respected, understood, and accepted—the kind of person who challenges you but also makes you feel safe. It's that kind of rapport that provides the foundation for the difficult and sometimes painful conversations that accompany most eating disorders. And it's those relationships that produce the conversations that make change seem possible. (2.)

People with eating disorders will often feel the same as you do: fearful that your relationship will be damaged by this problem. Eating disorders do cause a tremendous amount of stress and strain for everyone, and people need strong relationships to withstand that pressure. The thing most likely to get in the way of a supportive relationship is blaming. We'll help you protect your relationship by showing you how to avoid this pitfall. And since both of you are part of the equation, you'll both need to acknowledge that blaming yourself, the person with the problem, or anyone else won't help.

This chapter talks about where blaming comes from, how it works, how to end it, and how to replace it with something positive—respect.

WHY BLAMING STARTS

Most people like to figure out what causes problems, because they assume finding fault is the first step in fixing the problem. However, think of a plane crash: Knowing what caused the plane to go down won't change the outcome. The plane is wrecked. Figuring out what causes eating disorders is useful for psychologists who want to establish prevention programs and for doctors who need a clear appreciation of the physiology involved. But it's not very useful for people trying to cope with the everyday concerns associated with eating problems.

It's easy to see why people get caught up in the endless finger-pointing that accompanies most eating problems. We live in a culture that likes quick answers, and placing blame gives the illusion of being an instantaneous fix for the complex problems associated with eating disorders. Newspaper articles with headlines like "Mothers Responsible for Their Children's Finicky Eating," "Father Hunger: Dieting Daughters," and "Single Moms, Obese Children" all support the assumption that someone other than the person with problems is responsible.

Watching someone slide into a deeper and deeper hole with an eating problem is excruciatingly painful. In situations like these blaming begins innocently enough. Let's suppose:

- You are Ann's partner and you know that she spends her afternoons going from one fast-food restaurant to another, stopping only long enough to vomit in specially selected gas station bathrooms. You think, *How pathetic is that; doesn't she have any self-control?*
- You are Bob's brother, and he made you promise not to tell anyone that he cuts himself with a razor whenever his calorie count for the day doesn't match the goal he set for himself. You know he is training for a marathon but you can't stop thinking, *If anything bad happens to him, I'll never forgive myself.*
- You are a friend of fifteen-year-old Emily, who exists on less than 300 calories a day. She isn't menstruating and refuses to go to school because she "doesn't like it there." It's normal to think, *Where is this girl's mother, and why doesn't she do something?*

- You are Caitlin's sister, and she told you she can't keep food down ever since Max, her husband, told her she was looking a little chunky. You think, *That idiot turned her into a bulimic.*

In these scenarios it's easy to understand the need to place the blame somewhere, whether on yourself (particularly when you are a parent), or the person with the eating disorder (especially when you think she should know better), or someone else (when you think that another person is aggravating the problem).

However, as you may have already noticed, blaming yourself will make you miserable! Blaming others will make you angry, and make them defensive. And blaming the person with the problem will make him more secretive and less likely to talk to you. The end result is always repeated blaming, countless justifications, and angry words. Most important, with blame there are no winners and certainly no solutions.

In short, blaming inflames the problem.

HOW BLAMING WORKS

Blaming shuts down productive conversation about eating problems because it makes people defensive and muddles the question about who is responsible for change. Professionals and families all point their fingers when someone with an eating problem doesn't get better quickly. It is quite common to have parents mad at professionals, professionals mad at one another, and friends blaming family and the professionals.

Let's take a look at how blaming got in the way of finding solutions for the Fox family. Jason Fox, an attorney with a busy practice, was disturbed by the conflict between his very thin wife, Karen, and his slightly overweight sixteen-year-old daughter, Hannah. Jason noticed that his ten-year-old son, Mike, was spending all his time in his room, and Jason assumed he too was fed up with the conflict between his mother and sister.

When Jason asked Mike why he didn't want to come to the dinner table, Mike said, "Dad, you have no idea how sick I am of listening to their food fights. It's even worse when you're not here. Hannah eats like a pig and Mom won't eat anything. Nobody cares about me."

Jason decided to ask his wife if she had noticed how Mike was avoiding the dinner table. Karen said, "Mike doesn't have a problem; Hannah is the one you need to do something about. She is eating so much; she'll end up being the brunt of everyone's fat jokes. If you would just spend more time with her, she'd feel more loved and then she wouldn't be eating like this."

Jason felt angry at being blamed for Hannah's overeating. *It's Karen's fault,* he thought. *She is skin and bones. Who'd want to be like her? No wonder Hannah eats so much; she doesn't want to be like her mother. If Karen would stop screaming at me and get focused on setting a better example, Hannah wouldn't be eating so much.*

Later on, Hannah came to her father and announced, "I can't stand Mom hovering over every bite I eat. She is making me crazy. Can't you get her to back off?" The next day during his commute to work, Jason caught the tail end of a radio show describing what can happen when mothers reject their daughters for being overweight; rejection can lead a young woman to become promiscuous. Jason panicked and decided to speak to his doctor.

Dr. Wright, their family physician, didn't have much time to talk when Jason came for his physical exam, but he wanted to help.

Dr. Wright was aware of Karen's and Hannah's potential for health problems. He was worried about the fact that Karen's weight was low. He had treated her for a stress fracture in her foot last summer, even though she was only forty-three, he suspected that she might be showing early signs of osteoporosis. During her last physical exam, he talked with Karen about how thin she was, but she just smiled. Karen assumed he was giving her a compliment, and Dr. Wright didn't press the issue. When Hannah had her last physical exam, he noticed Hannah's weight gain and he was worried. So he said, "You're putting on the pounds, Hannah; you know the boys won't like that." Hannah blushed and didn't say anything but felt terrible.

Dr. Wright believed that children's problems would all be solved if their mothers stayed at home and attended to them "properly." He put it like this to Jason: "Look! You have to step up to the plate here and tell Hannah to understand that her mother is right to be concerned—being overweight is unhealthy. Then you need to tell Karen to quit her job as an aerobics instructor. Besides, she's too thin, anyway; tell her to put on some weight and Hannah will be just fine." When someone like Dr. Wright is pressed for time, you can see how blaming gives him the illusion that he is helping without really helping.

Nonetheless, Jason thought, *Okay, then, I'll go home and tell them what the doctor said.*

His conversation with Karen started and ended badly. "Karen, you've got to do better; you are driving Hannah into being a fat kid who will probably end up promiscuous because she has to get affection somewhere and you aren't giving her what she needs." Karen started to cry and left the room without answering. Jason couldn't understand why Karen wasn't more receptive to his comments.

His conversation with Hannah was also poorly timed and not helpful. Hannah was talking to her friend Sarah on the phone when her dad said, "I'd like to talk to you." Hannah pleaded, "Later, Dad; I'm on the phone."

"*Now,* Hannah." Jason said.

Hannah hung up the phone, turned to her dad, and said, "*What?*"

"I'm trying to make time for you, but all you do is talk to your friends; your mother is worried about your health, and if you would just be nicer to her she wouldn't get so upset."

At this point, Hannah had no idea how to deal with either of her parents. Her mother blamed her for being fat, and her Dad was blaming her for upsetting her mom.

She turned to her high school English teacher. She wrote in her class journal that her parents were fighting all the time because she was too fat.

Mrs. Sand, Hannah's teacher, was stupefied. She thought Hannah was talented and beautiful, so she was furious that Hannah's parents would make her feel fat. She assumed Hannah's parents didn't pay enough attention to how gifted Hannah was at writing. She blamed Hannah's parents for undercutting Hannah's confidence, and discussed this problem with the school guidance counselor, Mr. Thompson.

Mr. Thompson tried to talk to Hannah about the reasons for her self-esteem issues. He went up to Hannah during study hall and said, "Hannah, your teacher said you were worried about your weight. Girls your age are at such risk for eating problems, and your parents seem to be making this worse for you. If you are feeling bad about yourself, I'd be glad to set up an appointment."

Hannah was stunned. She felt invaded because now it seemed like everyone was worried about her weight. She didn't even know Mr. Thompson, and she did not appreciate his making assumptions about her or her family. She blamed her teacher for putting him up to it, and that made her angry.

What's so typical about this scenario is how all the people involved start blaming each other. Hannah blames her mom for criticizing her. Jason blames Karen for making Hannah neurotic. Karen blames Jason for not being more concerned about Hannah's weight. Dr. Wright blames the whole family for not subscribing to more traditional values. Hannah's teacher and counselor blame both parents for not getting along and for undercutting Hannah's confidence. In fact, there is so much blame in this situation that everyone feels helpless. No one offers any useful advice on how to identify the problem or, more important, how to talk about solving it. Even if neither Karen nor Hannah had a full-blown eating disorder when these fights got started, it is easy to see how these problems could escalate not only into eating problems but also serious family problems.

Most eating problems take on a life of their own. What gets them going in the first place is not usually what sustains them. In the example of the Fox family, Hannah's overeating probably began as a method of feeling better, full, nourished. Karen, feeling alarmed, grew more rigid in her own diet and exercise routines, hoping to influence Hannah to change. Because her mother's assumptions did not match Hannah's understanding of what was happening to her, their conversations ended in arguments—the inevitable outcome of blaming. It is easy to see that as each person blames someone else, everyone gets defensive, and they then fight with each other instead of working together to understand and then solve their problems.

PUTTING AN END TO BLAME

Blaming confuses responsibility. It is important to accept that:

> *The person with the eating disorder is*
> *responsible for his or her self-care.*

Blaming is like lighting a match to the worry and frustration most people experience when dealing with eating problems. Blame creates a focus of attention for all the pressure, strain, and tension we feel when we are helpless to control someone else's destructive behavior. But blame always leads to defense. When we blame, the person we blame will feel a need to justify and so will list all the reasons why his course of action was necessary. And in turn, he is likely to blame someone else, leading to an endless cycle of blame and justification. What will be missing is any reasonable accountability or responsibility for change.

It's even natural to defend yourself against your own blame with a vicious cycle of self-criticism followed by self-justification with a stream of excuses. That kind of internal conflict is stressful. Even though you promise yourself that you'll stop blaming, it's hard not to fall back into the trap. Being human, you will get frustrated with yourself, with others, and with the person who has the problem. Moreover, others will probably get angry with you.

Here are some suggestions you can use both to stop yourself from blaming and to persuade others not to blame you.

1. Acknowledge that your worries are *your* responsibility.
   - Blaming someone for making you worry will only make him feel guilty and defensive, and your blaming will fuel your anger.
   - It is not up to someone else to stop you from worrying. There are productive ways to channel your worries. Reading this book is a great place to start.
2. Resist the temptation to proclaim what someone else should do.
   - The urgency of witnessing someone hurt herself creates

pressure for action. But pushing for action will feel like criticism to the receiver.

- People intensely dislike making loved ones disappointed or angry, and so avoid those people if they fear they're going to be accused or blamed.

3. If blaming has already started, call a truce.
    - Pushing people to accept blame for what they have done wrong only makes them feel worse. In addition, since they can't undo the past it won't help to dwell on it.
    - Instead, use language that conveys you want to make peace, such as, "I'm feeling defensive and I don't like being in this position, especially when Vonda is in such trouble," or "I don't want to make up excuses for why I did what I did. Let's see if we can figure out what to do."

4. Try not to take it personally when others blame you. However, you will need to protect yourself from other people's anger, especially when you are already blaming yourself. Try to deflect this blame with comments like:
    - "Getting angry with me won't help. Let's try to figure out what we can do to make progress with this problem."
    - "I can see you're angry. My intentions are to help. Help me understand what we can do in the future."
    - "I can see you think this is my fault. I don't think so. Maybe we'll just have to agree to disagree. Meanwhile, let's work on what we can do to make this better."
    - "I'm worried too, and I wish we could focus on what we can do about this."

5. Overcome your own defensiveness and be willing to say, "I'm sorry!" Doing this can build trust between you and the other person.
    - Remember that a simple apology is best, and that you don't have to cut off your arm because you have made a mistake. Likewise, don't ask someone else to continue to apologize once a mistake has been acknowledged.
    - If you have blamed someone already, acknowledge the error. Try saying, "I realize I'm blaming you; I don't want to

do that," or "I can see I'm making you defensive; I didn't mean to put you on the spot."

6. Focus your attention on problem solving. You'll need to catch yourself pointing fingers. Notice when you are on the verge of saying:
   - *She should know better.*
   - *He needs to stop___.*
   - *If it were me, I would have ___.*
   - *He's making her___.*

   Try substituting these words:
   - *She has her reasons.*
   - *Since I'm not her, it's hard for me to know for sure why she decided to ___.*
   - *Even though he's doing ___, we still need to figure out what to do now.*

7. Nudge yourself to refocus on the positive.
   - Blaming someone for mistakes can blind you to the many more positive characteristics she possesses. Remind yourself of what you appreciate.
   - It's these positive aspects that will help you establish a productive course of action.

8. Try not to overanalyze. Even experts rarely know exactly what causes an eating disorder.
   - Trying to figure out what caused the problem in the first place will inevitably result in endless analyzing without the benefit of useful resolution. These circles of speculation, accusation, justification, and reanalyzing are draining. Practice saying, "I don't know why this happened," and see how much better you actually feel.
   - You can stop others from analyzing by pointing out, "I'm tired of this topic. I feel like I'm going around in circles; let's talk about something else," or "I guess we'll never know for sure why this happened. I'd rather focus on what we're going to do."

9. Leave the past in the past. Most of us have been blamed and felt guilty for things that can't be undone. Even when we're

sorry, we can't undo what is already done. All we can do is learn from our mistakes and even from the mistakes of others.

In short, it's easier to focus on providing support, setting limits, and problem solving when people aren't blaming each other. And it's easier not to blame each other when there is a climate of respect.

CULTIVATING RESPECT

Getting out of the blaming racket often leaves us with the feeling, "Okay, now what? What *can* I do?" You can cultivate respect.

We all want to feel that our choices and our opinions are respected, even when those we care about disagree with what we are choosing. Being respectful involves accepting that we do not have the right to control another person's choices even when what that person is choosing is harmful. Most of us know that we can't *force* people to quit smoking; we also can't force them to eat in a manner that we believe would be healthy.

And since the only real control we have is over ourselves, that's the best place to start. Value your peace of mind. Manage your own emotions as reasonably as you can. When you shift your thinking from controlling others to taking control of yourself, you will find yourself more in balance, and your confidence in handling these problems will grow. The combination of self-respect and respect for others will help you discuss the difficult issues that surround most eating problems. This section talks about how to do that.

MEETING PEOPLE WHERE THEY ARE

The first step in creating a respectful environment is acceptance. People often think that accepting what is happening is the same as approving of it. It isn't. As difficult as it may be to do, accepting that there are things *you cannot change* really matters. You will need to remind yourself of this fact many times.

Many of you reading this book are in a position of authority, such as a parent, a teacher, a coach, or a minister. Some of you may be friends, siblings, partners, or roommates, who, because of your relationship, do exert some influence over the person who is suffering with an eating disorder. It's easy to see why you would be tempted to use your influence or authority to push for changing behaviors, especially since you are convinced that the course you want is right. But this can backfire.

Take Larry. His son Kevin, a wrestler, has an eating disorder. Many wrestlers go for days without food, take laxatives, and avoid water in an attempt to meet coaches' or trainers' expectations. But Larry was stunned when, even after wrestling season was over, Kevin continued to take laxatives in an attempt to control his weight. Larry screamed, grounded, demanded, and in general made every possible attempt to force Kevin to stop this practice.

It didn't work. Why? Because Larry wasn't respecting his son. Before he could have a chance of establishing a meaningful dialogue with his son, something he really wanted, he had to start by accepting that Kevin was making his own choices. Granted they were choices he didn't like, but they were *his son's choices.* Accepting that the person you care about has the right to make his or her own choices is the first step in establishing a dialogue.

Lattelle faced a similar situation after her father died a long, slow death from brain cancer. She started to worry about her mother. She was horrified as she watched her mother eat compulsively. She knew her mom was depressed, but she was frustrated with her mother's complaints of an aching back and no social life. Furthermore, her mother wouldn't consider getting help for her depression. She told Lattelle, "It's only been six months since your dad died; I'm entitled to be depressed."

Her mother sat in front of the TV night and day and ate and ate and ate some more. Her blood pressure was dangerously high, which was all the more alarming to Lattelle because both of her mother's parents had died of strokes in their sixties. Lattelle was convinced she had to force her mom into action. So on her last visit, she turned the TV off in the middle of her mom's favorite show and insisted they go for a walk. When her mom refused, Lattelle blew up. "You are killing yourself with all this stuff you eat." She walked into the kitchen and threw the bag of chocolates her mom was savoring into the garbage disposal.

The more Lattelle monitored her mother's eating, tried to cajole her into exercising, or hounded her about seeing a therapist, the more defensive her mother got. Finally in desperation she asked Lattelle to just leave her alone, even though she really wanted her daughter close. It was easier for her mother to turn to her own sister for support. Lattelle's aunt accepted that her sister was grieving. She didn't approve of how she was coping, but somehow she managed to accept it. In contrast, Lattelle couldn't accept her mother's choices and so she criticized and bulldozed.

Lattelle's mom told her sister that the more her daughter pressed for change the more convinced she was that resting and eating were signs of her internal strength. She saw these behaviors as a strategy to take care of herself after having been so responsible for her husband's care while he was sick. She was tired of doing what was expected, and she decided it was better for her not to feel so obligated. Sometimes she would acquiesce to Lattelle's wishes, but only to get her daughter off her back. As soon as she wasn't monitored, she went back to doing what she liked, eating and watching TV.

Why was this? Lattelle's approach made her mother feel defensive, and so she resisted changing. However, her sister's acceptance created a feeling of safety so she could question herself and her self-destructive behavior. Lattelle's mother put it this way: "Arguing with my daughter made me defend what I was doing, so I couldn't begin to think about taking better care of myself. Talking to my sister made me dig deeper to think about what I was doing. That led me to stop bingeing."

FOCUSING ON THE WHOLE PERSON, NOT JUST THE EATING DISORDER

People with eating disorders are preoccupied twenty-four hours a day with food and with getting rid of their calories, fat grams, and carbs. This fixation makes it seem as if they have become nothing more than their eating disorder, because that is what we are focusing on in our minds too. For example, think of how often we call someone an anorexic instead of a person with anorexia. This label isolates them from the rest of us. Once they are branded with this title, it's easy for us to lose sight of their basic needs, rights, and other characteristics.

Also, all the things you like about someone can get lost when you are trying to change him, especially when you assume you know how, why, and when he should change. Accepting a person's right to choose her own coping style, her right to make her own mistakes, and, most important, her right to make changes at her own pace are essential ingredients for a respectful relationship.

That doesn't mean you should walk away. Quite the contrary. Your friend or loved one needs you to show interest in her full range of attributes and activities. Remind yourself of what you appreciate about her, and share the activities that you both like. Likewise, you want to make sure that you are listening, laughing, and sharing your feelings. You want to make sure that you continue to do all the things that made your relationship successful before she developed an eating disorder. Even when someone's behavior is at its worst, it's a good idea to make yourself available for the things you used to do before this problem took hold. Forcing participation will be a disaster, but offering invitations is supportive.

It's important that the person who is struggling senses your respect. He is more likely to appreciate your respectful intentions to be supportive and helpful if you can say, "This situation isn't your fault. I don't blame you for it, and you certainly shouldn't blame yourself either."

Taking blame is not the same as taking responsibility. It doesn't confer strength. It doesn't boost energy. It doesn't propel one forward. If you can take blame out of the equation, you will free the person you care about to look at where he is now and where he wants to go next. When you say you don't blame him, you express your belief in him and help him tap into his respect for himself. The real question is whether he wants to continue this way or whether he wants to change things. It's his call.

Let him know you are looking forward, not back. The past is past. Gone. Done. And what happens next is up to him. Be direct. Be matter-of-fact. That shows respect. The people you care about are more likely to sense your respect when you can:

- accept that the person with the eating disorder is responsible for her choices (we will deal with parental responsibilities in the

chapter on children), and that how you manage your worries is your own responsibility
- conclude that blaming won't help
- stop yourself from (overtly) criticizing others
- remind yourself and others that you are not to blame
- acknowledge that you cannot force solutions unless it's medically necessary (which we'll cover in the last section on emergencies).

Once the blaming stops and people work on cultivating respectful relationships, you can go back to enjoying each other and having a fulfilling relationship. And your support is more likely to help.

Change is one thing; progress is another.

∞—BERTRAND RUSSELL

Chapter Two

Understanding Change

∞

We often assume that what is evident to everyone else is evident to the person suffering with an eating disorder. We like to believe that stating the obvious—"This behavior is dangerous to your health!"—will lead someone to say, "I know I have to stop _____: overeating, vomiting, bingeing, avoiding eating, overexercising, and hating my body."

We're all tempted to start conversations about eating disorders by saying things like

- "Quit that."
- "Stop vomiting."
- "Eat more."
- "Eat less."
- "You shouldn't cut weight like that."
- "Trust me. You're beautiful!"
- "Stop dieting. You're *not* fat!"

But if telling people what to do really worked, there would be no smokers and there certainly wouldn't be any eating disorders.

UNDERSTANDING MOTIVATION FOR CHANGE

Your expectations for what needs to happen next will certainly influence what you want to say. But when your hope doesn't match someone else's readiness to change, all discussions of the eating disorder are likely to go poorly.

Conversations about eating problems fail for three fundamental reasons. First, the person with the problem may *not have defined* her behavior as a problem. Second, even if she does think she has a problem, she may *not feel ready* to make a change. And third, she may *not know how* she can make changes. In other words, she hasn't decided on the best way to make changes without suffering too many negative consequences.

Consequently, when well-intended people push for action before the person they want to help is ready, the inevitable result will be *resistance and defensiveness*.

Think about the last time you made some significant change. Perhaps you decided to get married, quit smoking, get divorced, move, get therapy, or change jobs. More than likely, it didn't *just happen* one day. Rather, you slowly realized the need for change. Then you thought about the pros and cons of doing something or nothing. Then you thought about possible ways to make "it" happen, and finally you did something. Most of us think about change as being only that action we decided to take one day. But really, it's what comes before the day we finally make the change that most often determines whether the outcome is successful. We are more apt to be successful if we carefully consider beforehand how we will handle temptations, setbacks, obstacles, stressful events, and all the other things that undo our best intentions. And then, in order to maintain progress, you have to figure out how to follow through. Since you'll want to motivate change and not inspire resistance, you'll need to gear your conversations toward that end.

The five stages that people suffering from eating problems typically go through as they attempt to change are:

- Precontemplation: Denying that there is a problem
- Contemplation: Reviewing the pros and cons of changing
- Preparation: Knowing there is a problem; not knowing what to do
- Action: Having a clear plan to tackle the problem and making the change
- Maintenance: The problem is better; progress needs to be maintained

Psychologists James Prochaska, John Norcross, and Carlo DiClemente have carefully sketched out these stages of change. (3.) Their original work was in studying people who quit smoking, but they have expanded their model to cover many other problems in their book *Changing for Good*. Their research, along with that of many other mental-health professionals who followed up on their original ideas, have inspired both changers and helpers. As we look more closely at each stage, we'll help you increase your effectiveness by outlining how you can gear your comments and strategies to someone's readiness to change.

STAGE ONE—PRECONTEMPLATION: DENYING THE PROBLEM

This is the hardest stage for most of us to deal with, because people in this stage are so defensive. They are not ready to consider that their eating is causing them problems, so they will rationalize, make excuses, and minimize the negative consequences of what they are doing. Typically they are annoyed when other people express their concerns.

It helps to remember that their unique justifications make sense to them.

- I can eat what I want. (Unsaid, but underneath it all—"I can always throw it up.")
- I'm not really hungry, so it doesn't matter that I'm not eating.
- These muscles are fabulous; who cares how I got them?
- I'll lose this weight; I've done it before.
- I've already broken my diet, so I might as well go for all the foods I want.
- I'll start over tomorrow.
- Laxatives relieve this pressure: I can't stand feeling so full.
- I'll gain weight if I eat fat, sugar, or white starches.
- I'll get fat if I don't count calories, fat grams, and carbs.

The individuals you want to help may realize that others would not endorse their logic. They might even say, "I know I shouldn't. . . ." However, if you listen closely, you'll hear the *but*; the common thread that runs through all their reactions is, "But I'm not ready to give it up yet." Even though they might wish for things to be miraculously different (such as being a normal weight and being able to eat whatever they want), they aren't ready to change. So they:

Blame their problems on circumstances:
- "I didn't have time to eat."
- "My stomach just feels sick when I eat, so I have to throw up."
- "You have to die of something, so I might as well keep eating."

Blame others:
- "My wife keeps baking me cookies; I can't hurt her feelings."
- "My husband will leave me if I'm not thin."
- "My kids will eat only junk food, so I do too."

Sound annoyed:
- "Look, what I eat is my choice!"
- "You're too critical!"
- "Stop trying to control me."
- "Quit nagging!"

Feel guilty:
- "I can't ___."
- "I'm not strong enough to ___."
- "I always fail."
- "Trying never works for me."

During this stage people don't see the need to make changes *now*. They justify their symptoms with complicated explanations for why they should be allowed to continue doing what they are doing. During this stage it's almost impossible to convince someone that change is possible. Whether overeating or undereating, people in this stage are more than willing to tolerate the negative aspects of their disorders, because their symptoms appear to them as necessary as breathing.

People in this stage steadfastly defend their right to do as they please, and the more you try to push them, the more likely you are to help them build better defenses, which feel like walls that keep you out. One of the best explanations for what it feels like to try and talk someone with anorexia out of their self-destructive behavior was described by Dr. Kelly Vitousek during a workshop on the treatment of eating disorders. She pointed out that talking to someone with anorexia is like trying to talk your seventeen-year-old daughter out of her dreadful boyfriend. (4.) People with eating disorders in the precontemplation phase defend themselves like teenagers in love.

So what can you do? During this stage issuing ultimatums, cajoling, confronting, or intervening rarely work. Avoid saying:

- "What you are doing is ridiculous!"
- "You're killing yourself."
- "You have to stop . . . (fill in the blank)."

What would be most helpful? First of all, look for openings to raise questions or plant ideas without insisting or pushing. Instead ask him to consider an alternative. For example:

- "You seem uncomfortable. I wish you would consider seeing a doctor."
- "You're graduating from high school. Maybe it's time to change some habits that are getting in your way."
- "That hike was really hard for you. What's up?"
- "You never eat with us. I don't understand why."
- "You seem so withdrawn. Is there anything I can do?"

While you'll probably get excuses to each and every one of these statements, at least you have brought up the issue without cornering the person you want to help. This helps because your expressions of concern plant the seed that something isn't right. That's why it is better just to say—briefly—what you are concerned about and why. Keep in mind how pushing can backfire.

Consider that they are probably looking to confirm their own position, even if they look compliant.

For example, Darsh's coach observed that he was overexercising and undereating. His coach told him that he had to see a counselor if he wanted to continue wrestling. But when he went for counseling, Darsh maintained he was fine and that his coach always overreacted to things. When his coach asked about his counseling session, Darsh said, "The counselor said I was fine and that you should lay off."

Rather than pushing for the counseling option (an action strategy), Darsh's coach would have done better to simply voice his observations and to maintain his support. For example: "Darsh, I've noticed how much you are exercising, way more than others on the team. Are you aware of how this can wear you down? Do you think that might be happening to you?"

Be willing to point out what you observe several times. Voice your concern and never demand agreement.

When people are in this stage and resistant to direct feedback, it's sometimes useful to describe the problems of other people who have successfully attempted change. "Remember Greg? He finally stopped his strict diet and now he is winning meets." Comment on how the eating disorder was hurting this person and how much strength it must have taken to tackle this problem.

STAGE TWO—CONTEMPLATION:
WEIGHING THE PROS AND CONS

During this stage people are considering options. They have some awareness that their behavior might be problematic. But the key words here are "might be." They feel divided. On the one hand they believe that what they are doing is necessary, and on the other they are often worried about the consequences of their eating behavior. They're like someone on a trapeze: One moment they are on one side; then the next time you see them they are on the other side. They know that eventually they have to stop on one side or the other—they can't stop in the middle. Essentially, they are weighing the pros and cons of each side.

Typically the pros are things like:
- "I like feeling in control."
- "People notice me."

- "I like being thinner than everyone else."
- "As long as I'm fat, my husband doesn't demand sex."
- "Because I purge, I can eat what I want."
- "If I eat regular meals, I'll gain twenty pounds in a week."

The cons are typically things like:
- "I wish I didn't think about food and calories all the time."
- "I'm sick of diet pills and laxatives."
- "I wish I could enjoy what I eat without worrying."
- "I hate my body; it keeps me from . . ."
- "I'm tired of this."

Because people are torn between two sides, their behavior is confusing. Those close to them often feel pulled in and then pushed out.

When someone is in this stage the most important thing you can do is listen and to support the thinking that is in favor of positive change. This is easier said than done. It is so painful to watch someone constantly teetering on the edge. But, even though the one you care about isn't ready for change *yet,* there is still a lot you can do that will be helpful—especially when you realize that the person you wish would change is profoundly torn about taking those steps.

When they say they are uncertain, you can:

Help them anticipate the consequences of not changing.
- "What do you think will happen if you don't change?"
- "Do you think not changing will be worse than changing?"
- "If you make these changes, what do you think will happen?"
- "Can you imagine how you will feel if . . ."

Get them resources that discuss their problem.
- "I saw this great film; would you like to see it?"
- "I read an article about what you were talking about."
- "My friend Alicia read this book on ___. Should we look at it together?"

- "My cousin tried ___. Would you like me to get some information about it from her?"
- "Another student of mine last year had this problem, and she decided to ___."

Reassure them of your concern and involvement without taking over.
- "Whether or not you change, I will still care."
- "I know this seems hard, but you'll eventually figure out what to do."
- "What have you thought about doing, and how can I help?"

STAGE THREE—PREPARATION: FIGURING OUT WHAT TO DO

During this stage the person is primarily considering what might be the best course of action. It's very important to remember that she isn't ready to actually change anything.

This stage can be frustrating to watch because you're more than ready to see something start to happen. But the person with the eating disorder is trying to find the right strategies so that she can follow through. At this stage she is now clear that the problems of maintaining her disorder outweigh her fears of making changes. She is apt to say things like:

- "I have to do something; I'm tired of this."
- "I can't stand it when people tell me I'm too thin."
- "I'm sick of feeling sick."
- "No one knows how miserable I am."
- "I have to stop pretending I'm okay."
- "This isn't good for me."
- "I've got to do something about this."

It is now that she is most open to suggestions and information about reasonable strategies for change. So long as you refrain from pushing her into action, it's okay to offer advice on what might work.

Listening to someone in this stage is also frustrating because the person with the eating disorder isn't actually doing anything different. And when the person who is struggling picks up on that frustration, it can make her defensive and move her backward. So instead of using her energy to move forward she is expending it on avoiding people who seem frustrated with her.

- "I told my daughter I wasn't vomiting but I still am, so now I can't face her."
- "I promised my coach that I would eat breakfast, but I can't make myself, so I lied. When he found out, I blew him off."
- "My wife thinks I'm not trying, and she gets so mad when I cheat on my diet, so I try to avoid her, and if I have to talk to her I tell her to quit nagging."

During this stage, it is important to provide support for getting ready to change without demanding any actual change.

- "It's great that you are thinking about taking better care of yourself. I'm happy for you."
- "You've got some great ideas about what to do—what do you think will work best?"
- "You seem happier now that you seem ready to move on this."
- "What's your next step?"
- "A lot of thought has gone into this; you've got a lot of courage to face this."
- "I support you; how can I help?"
- "What do you think will work? I'm glad to be a sounding board for your ideas."
- "This takes time; please be patient with yourself."

If you want to offer action strategies that you don't think the person has considered, this is the time to do it. They are ready to hear about things that have worked for other people. They are usually open to suggestions in this stage, just so long as you don't demand they follow your advice. You need to be ready to hear that your ideas aren't going to work for them.

STAGE FOUR—ACTION: TRYING SOMETHING

Once someone has decided on a course of action, it's best *not* to offer more advice or conflicting strategies. You can be most helpful by offering encouragement for the course of action he has decided to take. Knowing that someone cares enough to ask how things are going often supplies the extra boost to keep trying. You can say things like:

- "How are you doing?"
- "Do you want to talk about this or would you rather we talk about something else?"
- "Your efforts inspire me to tackle my problems with ___."
- "I'm thinking about you."

Questions about how things are going are particularly useful because it helps him evaluate his progress. The challenge is not to make judgments about that progress and to offer plenty of support for mistakes and setbacks.

STAGE FIVE—MAINTENANCE: SUSTAINING PROGRESS

We will go into more detail in chapter thirteen about helping people who have already made changes. For now, it's important to remember that it's the rare person who thinks about change, plans for change, changes, and then is completely set.

After someone who has been struggling finally figures out how to eat more comfortably or exercise more reasonably, she's going to feel great. But the stresses and strains of life often make it hard to maintain those positive attitudes. A negative comment from a boyfriend, a critical parent who mentions a weight gain, an anticipated vacation that might require a bikini, a Christmas dinner, all can contribute to making it hard to stay with what works.

In reality most of us cycle in and out of good times and bad. Often during periods of stress we revert back to old harmful ways, like Kaila. She was bulimic until her senior year in college, when she got fed up with being obsessed with calories, fat grams, and exercise regimens. Vowing to give this up once and for all, she got counseling, saw a dietician, and attempted to eat regular and balanced meals. She found she could actually eat more than she thought without gaining additional weight.

But several years after college, when she was busy working and not able to exercise, she gained weight. She started restricting what she ate, skipping meals, and grabbing snacks. The more she skipped and restricted, the more she started bingeing and the more weight she gained. She cycled back to the contemplation phase (stage two), knowing that she was harming herself, but not sure she wanted to make changes.

Finally her thirtieth birthday rolled around and a close friend risked saying, "Kaila, you don't seem happy. You're cranky all the time, just like that time in college. I'm worried about you."

This opened the door for a supportive conversation about how Kaila had had the courage to change once before and most likely would be able to do it again. Her friend reaffirmed her support and willingness to listen. This moved Kaila into the preparation stage, and she decided to go back to regular meals and make more time for exercise. Kaila's friend joined her during the action phase by going on walks and offering encouraging statements like, "You're doing great!" "It's fun to have this time with you." "Call me anytime you need a boost; I'm delighted that you are doing something so good for you."

MOST IMPORTANT

What we all need to realize is:

- **If you try to talk about action strategies, such as getting professional help, before the person is ready for action, your conversations will fail.** The time for suggestions for specific action strategies is during the preparation phase.
- **People cycle in and out of stages before they find successful solutions.** Sometimes they revert back to the contemplation stage after having taken some action that didn't work out too well.
- **Don't worry about trying to decide which stage the person you care about is in.** If you're not sure, it's best to assume that he is in an earlier stage rather than a later one. People with eating disorders try to please those they care about by claiming they are ready for change before they actually are. Some of the most helpful conversations about eating disorders allow the person suffering to express the conflict he feels about changing.

- Most people with eating problems worry not only about weight gain; they also deeply fear alienating the people they care about. Anything you can say about your steadfast commitment to your relationship will help. Reaffirm that you respect her efforts to do better and feel better and that you care about what happens.
- You can help by being involved without forcing premature solutions. Give up any expectations of how long the person with this difficult problem should be in each stage or when he should be moving along. Your patience will be appreciated.

Worry never robs tomorrow of its sorrow; it only saps today of its strength.

∞—A. J. CRONIN

Chapter Three

Taking Control of Yourself—Setting Limits

∞

*I*t is just as important to be patient with yourself as it is to be patient with the person who is struggling. And part of that patience is in accepting your limitations and finding ways to bolster your own reserves. Most important is setting some limits so that the support you offer is part of your life—but doesn't become your life.

Why is this important? First, because you deserve to keep your life intact. Second, if you are completely depleted, how effective can your support be? So it is important for both you and the person who is struggling that you have boundaries.

What happens when you don't set limits? The most typical outcome is that the people who are trying to be supportive become tired, frustrated, and resentful. The people with eating disorders feel guilty about having problems and therefore causing those who care about them to suffer and worry. The fallout is that the relationship becomes a source of stress for both people instead of a source of help.

When you try to control what you cannot control, you will always feel out of control. Since watching someone you care about behave in self-destructive ways is excruciating, it helps to shift your focus in the direction of controlling what *you* do rather than trying to control what someone else does. Changing this perspective is challenging for most of us.

In this chapter we'll help you take four steps toward getting back in the driver's seat:

- Assessing your role
- Setting your limits
- Figuring out a way to talk about what you need
- Following through on your limits and taking the hit from what follows

ASSESSING YOUR ROLE

A fabric of interrelationships is what gives our lives depth and meaning. Your role as partner, friend, parent, child, teacher, or coach is essential. When people step out of their role it almost always creates problems for relationships. You've probably had the experience of someone trying to mother you when she wasn't your mother, or doctor you when she wasn't your doctor. Maybe you can remember how annoying that was. People with eating disorders inspire such intrusive interventions because they seem to need so much help, so we have to be especially careful not to step out of our role.

- Cindy, a middle school teacher, started packing a lunch for Lilly, a student she feared was anorexic. She worried that Lilly's family wasn't concerned enough after Lilly told her that the reason she wasn't eating was because her mom didn't have time to fix her lunch.
- Kissa analyzed her husband's overeating; she concluded that he binged when he was worried about work. So she put the family's cookies and treats in a padlocked box whenever he had a stressful meeting.
- Kameko, a resident hall supervisor, collected information from Cheryl's roommates every time Cheryl vomited. She wasn't sure what she was going to do with this information, but she believed she should have it—just in case.
- Maryanne's fourteen-year-old daughter, Erin, refused to eat with the family. Even though she had been divorced for three years and the dinner table was now a peaceful place, Maryanne

didn't feel that she could ask Erin to sit at the table because she feared it would bring back bad memories of all the fighting.

All of these people acted with the best of intentions. They wanted to help. But each one lost sight of her unique and special role.

- Cindy, the teacher, had stepped into the role of mother. She could have been much more effective staying in her role as a teacher. She could have tried telling Lilly that she was worried about her lack of energy and her inability to function well in class. She could have said:
  - "You seem so low; would you like to talk?"
  - "You've lost a lot of weight; I'm worried."
  - "I know you said your mother won't pack a lunch, but why can't you find something in the house to bring to school for lunch?"
  - "Your grades are slipping. I'm concerned because I know you can do better. What do you think is wrong?"
- Kissa was a concerned wife. She wanted her husband to feel better when he was having stressful days, but when she tried to analyze his overeating, she slipped into the role of therapist or dietician. Then she moved into the role of policewoman when she padlocked the goodies. She could have stayed in the role of a concerned wife by showing her love and confidence in her husband's strengths. She needed to reassure him that she would help when she could without telling him what to do with statements like:
  - "I love you and I want you to have good health."
  - "I'm sure you can figure out what to do."
  - "Let me know how I can help."
  - "Would it help to talk more about what is going on at work?"
- Kameko had stepped into the role of private investigator, with a vague idea that it would help Cheryl. However, all this investigating left Cheryl feeling gossiped about and scrutinized, which only made her more convinced that she was fat and ugly and needed to vomit. Eating disorders inevitably create stress. What

Kameko needed to do was wait and look for opportunities to bring up the stress Cheryl was under. Then Kameko could tell Cheryl things like:

- "You seem very stressed out. If you want help, I can tell you where to go."
- "I'm worried about ___, and ___. If you want to talk about this, I'm concerned and available."
- "A lot of students develop problems with food when they're under pressure. Do you feel like that's happened to you?"

- Maryanne needed to stay in her role as mom, not therapist. She needed to be the head of the household and feel comfortable saying things like:
  - "I expect you to be at family meals, whether or not you choose to eat."
  - "This is what we do in this family; we eat together on these days, and I expect you to be there."
  - "If this is too hard for you, we need to figure out why. Maybe we should consider therapy."
  - "I want you at the dinner table. Can you tell me why this is a problem for you?"
  - "I want you here and so do your brothers and sisters. Be here and be pleasant."

If you can be clear about what your role is, you are well on your way to feeling more peace of mind about what you can and can't do. And while it's easy to assume that being concerned means you need to step out of your role and do something right away to fix whatever you are observing, this strategy will fail.

We all know that doctors don't treat their own family members. Even more important, when you aren't a doctor, you don't want to step into that role. Remind yourself that you need to do what good spouses, parents, friends, coworkers, teachers, and coaches do when they are worried about people they care about. That is:

- Express concern about what you observe.
- Remain available.

- Be clear about your expectations.
- Share activities that are mutually enjoyable.
- Talk about the things that are important to each of you.

No matter what your role, here are some strategies that clearly won't work:

- Don't analyze motivations or intentions; in other words, don't try to be a therapist.
- Don't try to force someone to stop self-destructive behavior.
- Don't become a detective.
- Don't monitor someone else's eating, calories, or food intake.

DECIDING ON REASONABLE LIMITS

When you want to establish limits, consider first what you actually control. Very often people try to control things they have no control over. For example, Matt wished he could force his anorexic daughter, Saran, to eat. Matt was divorced from Saran's mother and they were on bad terms. He found it difficult to talk to Saran about anything without fighting.

When Matt called her, she was rude and demanding. The only conversation she seemed willing to have involved pleading with her father to buy her a car. She was sullen when they went out to dinner, refusing not only the food but also the conversation by answering all his questions with one-word answers. Matt wanted to set limits on what Saran ate, as well as on her demanding and rude behavior. Wisely, he came to terms with the fact that the only control he actually had was over himself. He could make Saran's anger a topic of conversation, he could limit the time he spent with her when she was rude, he could clarify with her how much money he was willing to spend and what that money could be used for; these were things he could control. He realized that what Saran ate was under her control.

So the kind of limits you set should be based on what you actually have control over. For most of us that means:

- How we spend our money.
- How we spend our time.
- Where we focus our attention.
- How we behave.
- What we choose to say.
- How we evaluate what's good for us.

Here are some general guidelines for setting those limits.

DON'T LET YOURSELF GET DRAWN INTO
ILLOGICAL THINKING

We know that people with eating problems will attempt to pull you into their distorted thinking. They will:

- Argue that their choices don't or shouldn't affect other people.
- Believe that vomiting is an effective means of weight control.
- Think that taking laxatives will help prevent calories from being absorbed.
- Assume that binge eating for years won't have serious consequences.
- Justify serial binges with assumptions like, "I won't do that again."
- Fail to recognize how their behavior has changed.
- Wish someone or something could make them perfect (i.e., thin enough).
- Presume that their diet rules must be honored by others at all times.
- Demand that others care but impose the rules for just how that care should be delivered.

You can avoid this "crazy" thinking by reminding the person you care about that you hold different views than they do about weight, dieting and exercise and that you can have a successful relationship even if the two of you don't always agree. Don't try to convince her. It's tempting but it won't work.

For example, Greg, who has an eating disorder, liked to ask his roommate José about everything José ate, and then Greg would add comments like, "Doesn't it bother you to eat all that at one time?" or "You mean you don't count your calories?" He also asked José questions about what Greg should eat, like "Do you think this is okay, or is it too much?"

When José said, "What you eat is your choice; it seems okay to me," Greg would argue back, "You don't really think it is okay because you ate less."

Fortunately, José didn't bite. Instead he said, "You'll have to decide what's right for you, but I don't want to get into these conversations with you. Let's focus on something else." In this way José took control of what he could control, namely what he talked about with his roommate. And he decided not to get drawn into these repetitive conversations that seemed so pointless.

DON'T LET YOUR ROUTINES BE CHANGED TO

ACCOMMODATE THEIR ROUTINES

When the person you care about asks you to eat more or less than you intend in order to make her more comfortable, you'll need to be clear that this is not reasonable. For example, Summer had stopped vomiting and bingeing, but she still had problems believing that her weight was normal.

Her boyfriend, Darnell, was stymied when Summer told him she wanted him to eat more, so that she wouldn't feel like she was eating too much. He worried that if he didn't eat he might upset her, maybe even start her back into bingeing and vomiting.

Finally Darnell spoke up and said, "Summer, I care about you, and no matter how much you eat, it won't make me care any less about you, but when you want me to eat when I'm not hungry so *you'll* feel better about your eating, I have to draw the line."

As a person concerned about someone with an eating disorder you'll need to:

- Eat when you are hungry.
- Eat in ways that make sense to you.
- Complain when someone has eaten all of the special foods you have purchased for yourself.
- Eat at the restaurants you enjoy.
- Not prepare special meals on a daily basis.

Don't Make Excuses for Someone Else's Behavior

Just because someone has an eating disorder, it doesn't mean she should be excused from the normal requirements of daily living. In fact, maintaining these expectations often helps the struggling person recognize that there is a problem that needs attention.

Beth, a mother of four teenage children, stopped cooking for her family when she became bulimic. She kidded herself into believing that her children wouldn't care if she didn't prepare dinner and that they could find something to eat on their own. She rationalized that they all had busy schedules, and that not cooking could allow her to avoid dinner squabbles among her children.

Her husband, Derek, was angry that the family dinner hour had evaporated. He enjoyed sitting down to a meal with the family and believed it was helpful in maintaining connections with his children. His schedule made it difficult for him to take on the cooking, but he did it anyway. Beth didn't eat with the family. Derek knew his wife was struggling, so he made excuses to himself and their children about why his wife was not only not cooking but also not eating with the family.

It is easy to understand why he didn't want the kids to know that their mother was secretly bingeing and vomiting. But the more Derek made excuses to the children, the more he got caught up in her irrationality. He started making excuses to friends for why they couldn't attend dinner parties. Eventually both Beth and her husband started to believe their laundry list of excuses:

- "She's got a stomach problem."
- "She isn't hungry."
- "She's too busy to eat."
- "She needs to be with the children, so we can't go to dinner."
- "She needs to work on this project; she doesn't have time for cooking."

All this covered up the fact that Beth had a serious problem.

Derek needed to realize that all these excuses were allowing Beth to ignore how she was neglecting her responsibilities to her family and friends. He might have said something like, "Beth, I feel like I've made a mistake. I've been making excuses for why you will never eat with people, when I know that what is really happening is that you are struggling with these eating problems. Can we talk about working on what is really going on?" Or, "I don't like making up excuses for you. It makes me feel like a liar. I don't think I can keep this up, but I'm worried about how it will affect you." And if he thought this might be time to bring up getting help he could say, "I might feel more like making an occasional excuse if I really thought you were seeking help. But since you aren't helping yourself, I feel like I'm making it easier for you not to get better."

Notice that Derek should not tell his wife what she should do or think but rather talk about himself and how he is feeling, and about what he is willing and not willing to do.

Stand Up for Yourself

Allowing yourself to be insulted or hurt will only set the stage for the destruction of your relationship. Don't stand by while the person you're worried about blows up at you, is irritable, or hurts you with hostile remarks. It's reasonable to expect normal, courteous treatment even though the person you care about is having a hard time.

Of course, you are acutely aware of the suffering and discomfort caused by the eating disorder, and this awareness can leave you feeling that you should always be available, supportive, and responsive no matter what. And you can end up feeling like a hostage—fearing that any upset or disagreement will lead to more disordered eating. Both of these are traps that will hurt the relationship you are trying to nurture. It is both kind and necessary to continue to expect reasonable treatment from the person who is struggling. For example:

- "You don't need to yell at me; I'm standing right here."
- "I'm not going to raise my voice. Can we talk about this calmly?"
- "I can see you are very angry (or upset). I'd rather wait to talk about this when we are both less angry (or emotional)."
- "I'm not willing to talk about this now."
- "Those remarks hurt. Are you trying to hurt me? What's up with that?"
- "I'm not going to continue this conversation; let's talk later."

Don't Give Up the Things That Are Important to You

You won't be happy if you give up valued activities or friends while you are trying to help someone. It is essential that you don't let someone's eating problems take over your life. You will not be able to stay involved if you don't keep up the activities you enjoy.

Remember, only *you* can make choices about what *you* need to do.

Leza was so terrified that her bulimic daughter was going to throw up that she followed her around after she ate. She quit going to her bridge group and didn't even go to work on days when her daughter was home from school. Leza's attitude was, *I'm her mother. How can I not devote all my time to my daughter's problem?*

But underneath, Leza was cultivating resentments that she was hardly aware of. One night she realized that she was furious that she wasn't able to do the things that had made her feel good. She missed her friends and their lively conversations. But she also realized that part of her feared that her friends would judge her, that they were thinking things like, *How come Leza can't get her daughter to stop being bulimic?* and, *If she were a good mother she would ___(fill in the blank).* Leza felt guilty. She knew that she was cutting herself off from the support she needed because of her fears of being criticized about being a good mother.

Leza needed to reach out and let her friends know that she was scared of their criticism. She needed to say:

- "I don't know what to do about my daughter's problems, and I'm afraid you'll judge me because of it."
- "Right now I'm getting so much advice from everyone. It helps to talk about something else."
- "I need to get my mind off all this trouble, and game night really helps. I'm so glad that I have a place to go where I can forget about what bothers me."
- "I'm too worried about my daughter to come this week, but this group is important to me. Please let me know what happened."

Another reason people resist telling their friends is because they feel disloyal to the person who has the problem. Meg's son was anorexic, and even though she knew his problems were obvious to others, she felt like it would be invading her son's privacy to talk about it. Kai was aware his friends knew his wife was obese, but he found it hard to talk about her decision to have bariatric surgery, about his fears that the surgery would harm her and that he would lose her. Both Meg and Kai ended up feeling alone and isolated.

The antidote to this isolation is to accept that your life, your fun, your fears, and your needs for distraction matter. And you need to accept that if you *don't* take care of yourself, you won't be able to help those who most need your assistance and support.

BE WILLING TO HAVE OTHERS GET ANGRY WITH YOU

When you set limits about what you will and won't do, you are apt to be met with resistance and anger. You need to be willing to "take the hit." This means recognizing that others may get angry when you stand up for what you need. Some people really make it hard, saying things such as, "You're awful!" or "You're the one making me sick." And going right for the heart: "You don't care about me." Anything to get you to back off.

Most people back off from setting the limits they need because they are worried that the person they care about will be angry or upset, and they fear this will make them sicker.

Families can come unglued making accommodations for someone with an eating disorder. They give up eating certain foods, change dinner hours, and stop going out together, all in the name of "help." Well, it won't help. If you make yourself miserable, you'll end up resentful. It's reasonable to set the limits you need to keep yourself sane. For example, you may need to say you can't receive phone calls after midnight or that you can't be disturbed when you are at work. It will help your relationship.

DON'T LET THEIR ANGER FUEL YOURS

When someone is angry with you, it's all too easy to say something that will boomerang—even if it's something that you think needs to be said; even if it's trying to get them to take responsibility and move forward. You may be tempted to say things that are better swallowed. These things can sound like blaming, or a threat to withdraw support, or as an unreasonable demand, or as if you think battling an eating disorder is easy.

HERE ARE SOME EXAMPLES OF THINGS TO AVOID SAYING AND WHY

When we feel out of control we are apt to make the mistake of trying to force compliance by blaming, finding fault and making demands. These tactics don't work.

"This is your fault. No one else's."

Maybe she's trying to blame you for her eating disorder, but it won't help to shift that blame back to her. Being blamed for things doesn't make anyone feel better, and it certainly doesn't help anyone feel strong. Instead of trying to assign fault for what has already happened, help her find the strength to take responsibility for what will happen next. Hopefully that will be a step toward recovery.

"How did you ever get yourself into this mess?"

You may think that by exploring how this came about you might be able to find a way to fix things. But what he will hear is that you think he brought this on himself and that you plan to put all his feelings and thoughts under a microscope. Figuring out what is driving the eating disorder is something professionals are trained to do, and can be important, but it's not the best role for you to play. Your role is to be supportive.

"Get control of yourself."

When we're worried and frustrated that things aren't going well, we can sometimes lash out without even realizing it. Yet if we stop to remember anyone saying these same words to us, we will realize how harsh they can feel to the person receiving them. In old movies when someone became hysterical she would get a slap in the face to shock her out of it. In real life this doesn't work, and neither does saying these words, which are the verbal equivalent of a slap in the face—and just as hurtful.

"I don't think I want to see you until you've taken steps to deal with this."

You are trying to get him to acknowledge that there is a problem. You are trying to give him an incentive to work on it. What he hears, though, is rejection. That you don't care enough to stick around. That you don't really enjoy being with him anyway. That he disgusts you. He may already feel bad about himself; he doesn't need to feel worse. He needs to hear expressions of your confidence in his ability to improve over time. Not seeing him will feel like rejection, particularly if he isn't able or ready to change just yet. That pressure will feel like manipulation and is apt to inspire resistance rather than progress.

"This is hurting everybody. Don't you care?"

Maybe you want to shock her into seeing beyond herself. Have the teenager see how this affects her younger siblings. Have a mother see how this affects her children. Have people who are suffering see how this affects parents, friends, partners. Some people who hear this will feel you are accusing them of being selfish. They will resent that and withdraw from you. Others will feel tremendous guilt at hurting others. If they don't accept that guilt, they will feel resentful. If they do accept the guilt, they will have a terrible burden to carry. Either way, the energy they need to battle their way back will be depleted, and their relationships with people who support them will be strained.

"What time will you be home? I expect you to come straight home from school/work."

From a parent's standpoint, from the point of view of the spouse or loving partner of someone with an eating disorder, this is an attempt to ward off eating-disorder behaviors. It is too easy to stop at a convenience store, load up on junk food, and binge in the car. It is too easy to stop at gas stations on the way home to purge. But you can't be in the car with the people you love wherever they go; you can't confine them to their rooms. They will find a way no matter what you do. It doesn't help if you reinforce a climate of hiding and sneaking around. That only fosters lies and manipulation and estrangement and silence. The recovery process thrives in an atmosphere of openness, acknowledgment, and support.

HOW TO TALK ABOUT SETTING LIMITS

Here are some suggestions for things to say that can open up the possibility for discussion.

"I wish I could fix everything for you, but I know I can't. I want you to know how much I care and that I believe in you."

When you say this, you show respect for her autonomy as a person. At the same time you acknowledge she is struggling with something that is very difficult.

"I love you, and it's hard for me not to charge right in. But I promise not to do that; I won't take over."

It's important to say this explicitly—that you recognize certain boundaries, that you recognize the difference between wanting to make things right for someone you care about and actually stepping in and making all the decisions. This can clear the air and set the stage for him to take positive steps.

And as he sees over time that you really haven't taken over, he will be more able to open up, share what is going on, and ask for appropriate help.

"Where you go from here is up to you. I'll be there to help when you think I can."

When you say this, you take away her need to resist you. Resistance takes up a lot of mental space and energy. It tends to make people hold on to what is and to stay wherever they are. The idea that what happens next is up to her—and that there is somewhere else to go—is liberating. It opens up possibilities. And it says that you respect that what she chooses to do, how she plans to get there, and, most important, when she decides to start are all up to her.

"There may be some things I can't do, because I have choices to make, too, and responsibilities to others as well as myself, but I'll be here, and support you, and help where I can."

Though sometimes people with eating disorders withdraw, at other times they can be very demanding. It's okay to set boundaries that protect you as well as them. And it is likely to help them, too. When we treat others with respect, we tend to respect ourselves more, too. That promotes the healthy sense of self a person with an eating disorder might have lost.

"I have the utmost respect for you and hope it always shows. I know you feel the same way about me. Sometimes, however, I feel you don't act that way. I don't know if it's part of the stress you've been under. Even so, it hurts. Please don't take it out on me; we can talk about these things without attacking each other or putting each other down."

It's usually not a good idea to let things fester. Someone with an eating disorder may lash out at you out of their pain and frustration. It's okay to let that go when it happens occasionally. We can understand that our friends are suffering and that they may lose it once in a while; after all, we've all done the same thing. But it's not a good idea to remain silent if it happens a lot or continuously. It can damage your relationship; it can become a habit for the person who is doing it; it can be a way to avoid dealing constructively with what is going on. In the end, you both lose. Bringing it up is an opportunity for you to become closer, to show each other mutual respect, and to give each other mutual support.

"It feels as if you've been avoiding me. Have I done anything to make you uncomfortable? If so, I'm sorry."

This lets him know you miss him. That he matters to you. That you're open to listening. It may also make him aware that he has made changes in his life without realizing it, or without consciously deciding to do so. And that might start him thinking about what's causing that.

"I wish I could do all the things you ask but it's too much for me. Let's talk and figure out which things we can do."

You may need to say "no" to some things—either because it's more than you can commit to or because there are things you feel would hurt her rather than help her. This is a way to say "yes" while saying "no." Yes, you want to be there. Yes, there a lot of things you can do. Yes, you can work together on this. When you are reasonable and forward-looking, you create an atmosphere in which possibilities exist.

They may forget what you say, but they'll remember how you made them feel.

Chapter Four

Conversation Basics—Maximizing the Impact of What You Say

∞

*T*oo often, what we intend to say doesn't come across as well as we had hoped. We try to offer support and get rejected for not understanding. We want to help, but are criticized for trying to take over. Some of us even end up being accused of causing more problems. We wonder where we went wrong and worry about what to do differently.

Fortunately, there are communication strategies that improve the effectiveness of difficult conversations. This next section lays the groundwork for effective communication by going over how best to approach some difficult topics.

HOW WE SAY IT—MAKING THE MESSAGE CLEAR

It isn't just the words themselves; it's *how* we say them. When we are upset, frustrated, tense, or very concerned, we focus so much on the way we are feeling that we don't always think about how our words sound. And the same words don't sound the same as they would if we were relaxed, calm, confident, at peace. It's a good idea to think about all the messages people get from the way we come across, messages we may not intend at all.

USING YOUR VOICE

The first thing that happens to many of us when we're upset is that we tend to speak much more loudly. That raises the temperature of the conversation very quickly, because the other person is likely to mirror your voice, get upset, and speak loudly, too. You may not be angry, but the loudness by itself will make it sound as if you are, and the person you are talking to will react to that more than to the words you say.

Another thing that happens is that we tend to talk a lot faster. When we speak very quickly, we make it hard for others to process what we're saying. And the speed conveys a lot of intensity, too, just as loudness does, which can make your words feel like an attack—a barrage of verbal bullets. You want the person you care about to be open to what you are saying; if it feels like an attack, he will only want to defend himself and justify his position.

The third thing we do is say too much. Less is more, especially when you are tackling a difficult subject and your audience is not receptive. If you talk quickly, loudly, and a lot, the person listening can feel as if what she has to say doesn't matter. Say a little bit and wait for a response. Talk slowly and calmly. Put your caring in your voice. Be matter-of-fact and warm. It's not enough for your words to be nonjudgmental; your voice has to convey that, too. If you're overwrought, you won't be able to do that, and you might push the sufferer away.

This is because tone of voice is a huge part of any message we receive. Studies show that when tone of voice conflicts with the words we hear, we tend to trust the tone of voice more than the words. The range of tones of voice is huge. There are probably as many tones of voice as there are moods and feelings, ranging from chilly to heated, from calm to tense, from ecstatic to inconsolable, from sincere to sarcastic, from helpful to hurtful, from bitter to forgiving, from flexible to rigid, from domineering to subservient, from respectful to degrading, from confident to timid, from distant to intrusive. Sometimes we want to convey one of these extremes—such as respectful, sincere, flexible— and sometimes we want to strike a note somewhere in the middle, such as between distant and intrusive. If you want tone to work for you, think about the positive feelings you have and those feelings will flow naturally into your tone.

USING YOUR EYES

Make sure you make eye contact, as you would in any other conversation. If you avoid looking at him when you speak, no matter how supportive your words, you will be sending a conflicting message. The person you are speaking to may interpret that in a number of ways: that you are embarrassed, that you no longer respect him, that you find the whole subject distasteful, that you are impatient with his behavior, that you're in a rush just to get this over with, or that you don't think of him in the same way any longer.

The expression in your eyes matters. The person you care about will meet your eyes and know if you are angry, fearful, sincere, uncomfortable, trusting, patronizing, solid, closed off, or meeting him halfway.

USING YOUR BODY

Don't turn your body away from her. We often do that to protect those we love when we are feeling deep emotion. For example, parents will do that so their children won't see their tears; in their attempts to be matter-of-fact and calm, they may fiddle with something as they talk or as they are listening to what their kids are saying. But instead of seeing protective, concerned behavior, kids think their parents aren't paying attention, or don't want to talk, or are so disappointed in them that they won't look them in the eye. They may even think it's a sign of rejection—that their parents don't love them anymore. By putting warmth and expectancy in your voice, by keeping the rest of your body language open, you convey interest and support. On the other hand, if you lean over her, she'll feel you are trying to take over; and if you cross your arms or legs, she might feel you are angry, set in your thinking, and not able to really hear what she has to say.

Sometimes touching her hand, arm, or shoulder can help you connect and convey caring. If you are sure the person you care about is comfortable with touch, this can be effective for you, too. It will help you relax; it will help you put yourself in that place where warmth, a slow pace, and openness will happen naturally. If it doesn't feel as if you are going on the offensive, she won't feel she needs to retreat, avoid, or attack in response.

Touch, though, is something to be particularly careful about when someone you know has an eating disorder. Their sensitivity to what they perceive as "problems" with their bodies can make them very leery of being touched. (More on that in chapter seven.)

LISTEN, LISTEN, AND THEN LISTEN MORE

If you want people struggling with an eating disorder to be open with you, you need to show you are willing to listen by waiting to hear what they have to say. And you need to give them your full attention. You might ask yourself how often you have ended up thinking, *I don't know why she said I wasn't listening. I heard what she said.* But hearing her words and truly hearing *her* aren't the same thing. Being on the receiving end of this criticism is especially painful when we think we are good listeners. However, most of us know when someone isn't listening intently, when his mind is drifting off, when he is working on something else, when he's dying to get a word in edgewise, when he wishes the conversation was wrapping up, when he is just plain bored with the interaction. And we know what it feels like. It feels like the other person isn't really there with us.

It is easy to underestimate how very difficult listening can be. The biggest obstacles to listening come when you are:

- **Trying to speak and listen at the same time.** You can't listen if you are planning what to say next. Our own thinking easily distracts us when we are focusing on the points we are going to make. Allow time for the other person to say whatever is on her mind without interruption. When you are sure that you do, in fact, understand what she wanted to say, then and only then should you figure out what to say in response. Be patient with yourself. Remember, it takes practice to break up the tasks of speaking and listening into two separate activities.
- **Feeling overwhelmed by strong feelings.** Watching someone grapple with an eating disorder can bring up very powerful emotions for those who are close by. It can leave us reacting

rather than listening. It helps to be aware of your own strong feelings and to recognize that those feelings are apt to distort what you hear. For example, if you are angry, you are more likely to listen for things that will justify your anger. That makes it harder to hear things that run counter to what you were expecting. Likewise, when you're afraid, you will pay attention to other things that make you fearful. Unfortunately, your fears could even get in the way of hearing the reassurances you are hoping for.

Since listening is more difficult than it might appear, it's a good idea to check out what you hear by paraphrasing or "mirroring" what you heard. Too often we say things like, "I understand," without explaining what it is we understand. It helps to make those perceptions clear and to *ask* the other person if you are understanding correctly.

For example:

> "Kara, I'm not sure I'm getting this right. You want me to stop asking you how you feel. You wish I'd talk about something else. Have I got it right?"
> *"You're close. I'm trying to tell you that I don't want to talk about my eating disorder!"*
> "Okay, so you don't want to talk about the eating disorder, but other feelings are okay to talk about?"
> *"Yes, that's right. Thank you for trying to understand."*

After you are clear that you understand what the other person was trying to convey, you could give your reaction to what was said:

> "I'll respect your wishes not to talk about your eating problems, but I want you to know that makes me feel closed out. I don't like feeling closed out, because I care about what is happening to you."

What we're describing is often called *active listening.* But you don't have to have training in "mirroring," empathic listening, or some other method of making sure that you understand what is being conveyed in order to listen well. Simply practice checking out what you heard by asking, "I think this is what you said; have I got it right?" This practice will help when you are talking about the many difficult issues surrounding most eating disorders.

Many people resist using these techniques because they think it sounds artificial. Of course, you don't want to sound like a parrot, but active-listening techniques show that you are trying to understand what the other person is experiencing. That kind of effort is generally appreciated. It is also essential to building the trust and safety that are necessary for another person to have confidence in your ability to handle tough topics.

And it will also help you. It's a lot more comfortable not to have to guess about whether or not you understand what the other person means to say. Feeling confused, wondering what he means, and thinking that he can't possibly believe what he is saying are all signs that you may need to check out your take on the situation. Actually, if you think there is any small chance that you may be misunderstanding, always ask, "Am I getting this right?" "Do you think I'm missing something?" or "What is it you would most like me to understand?"

REMEMBER THAT TIMING MATTERS

If you've ever dealt with real estate salespeople, you know that the three most important factors are "location, location, location!" Likewise, when you are trying to talk to someone about an important, sensitive matter, the three most important considerations are timing, timing, and timing.

We have all had the experience of bringing up an important issue in the middle of an argument. It's hard to resist the temptation to blurt out what you really think in the midst of a heated debate. Yet we all know this is likely to "blow it." When we want to communicate something important and want the other person to be open to it, timing matters most.

Remind yourself that you want what you say to be heard as you intended. This reminder is an essential step in the direction of thinking ahead and planning for the best way to bring up a difficult subject. *Don't approach a difficult topic* when the person you care about is:

- drinking
- tired
- doing something else that is important and apt to be distracting
- saying they don't want to talk now
- first getting up in the morning
- going to bed at night
- in front of other people

A compelling example of how not to bring up a difficult topic occurred one Halloween around midnight, when all the girls on the third floor of a college residence hall decided to confront a friend about her bulimia. They had all been drinking, and when the counselor arrived, she found six girls in costumes, sobbing and yelling. One of them explained, "We had to tell Ginny that we all know she's bulimic, and now she won't come out of the bathroom."

It took a while for her to convince them that it would be better to talk about this in the morning and to reassure Ginny that it was safe to come out of the bathroom.

You might be wondering when exactly is a good time to have a difficult conversation. Here are some better times to try a difficult conversation:

- When the person you are concerned about says she is ready to talk.
- When you have some privacy.
- When you won't be interrupted.
- When you have adequate time.
- When the other person is at his best (rested, comfortable, not distracted).

You might also consider it a good time to talk when you have:

- set aside some special time (after requesting a time to talk)
- confidence that you will be able to follow up in a few days

- clarity about what you want to say
- considered whether writing your concerns might be better, because it would give the person you're worried about time to react in private
- an awareness that not discussing these matters will affect the quality of your relationship.

It's often wise to trust your intuition. If your instincts tell you that this is the right time to bring up a difficult topic, it's worth a try. If you have any doubt, you can begin by asking if this would be a good time to talk. "I have something I want to talk to you about. Is this a good time?"

CHECK OUT YOUR ASSUMPTIONS

Thinking you know exactly what another person is going to say creates a mind-set that can distort what you hear. These distortions can lead you to misinterpret motives and intentions.

We often assume we know how others are feeling when we have gone through something similar in our own lives. It's easy to imagine that someone who is going through what we went through will react the same way we reacted. Unfortunately, this can significantly interfere with hearing that his or her experience and feelings are different from yours. It's better to assume that no two experiences are ever identical. Listening for the differences can help you communicate your understanding of another's unique circumstances and emotions.

We also tend to assume that we know what someone else is thinking, especially someone we know well. More often than not these assumptions become so automatic, we aren't fully aware of how much they influence what we say. It's important to check out assumptions. There is too much room for wrong ideas to grow if you don't.

Let's look at how this problem led to misunderstandings for John and Suzanne. Suzanne assumed that John was angry with her because he didn't ask her to his company's Christmas party. John wasn't angry; he was worried that Suzanne wouldn't want to go because it might interfere with her diet. But Suzanne, feeling defensive and convinced that

John had no right to be angry with her, retaliated by giving him a cold shoulder. Suzanne assumed that she knew what John was feeling, even though she didn't ask. John was aware that Suzanne was angry with him, but he assumed it was because he had bought another piece of exercise equipment. So he told her that he planned to take his new stair-climber back to the store. But Suzanne didn't care about the stair-climber; in fact, she was pleased that he was trying so hard to exercise. So she cut him off midsentence and left the house. All of these misunderstandings could have been avoided with a few well-placed questions about what was going on.

Many people develop automatic thoughts in response to someone's eating problems:

- She always blows her diets.
- He'll never change.
- She's going to the bathroom; she must be vomiting again.
- He won't wear that because he thinks he's fat.
- She won't go out to eat with us.
- He's trying to kill himself with food.

These basic assumptions are often communicated even when we are trying to hide what we think, particularly through our body language. Rolling eyes, sneering gestures, and long sighs convey vague negative messages that often undercut what we really want to communicate.

The people we're concerned about who have eating disorders also misinterpret *our* actions. They frequently assume we aren't telling them the truth, especially when we say things like, "You're not fat," or "I love all of you," or "It doesn't matter to me what we eat," or "I think you're beautiful inside and out." People with eating disorders assume we say these things because we have to, not because we really mean them.

Don't let these assumptions stay hidden. Bring them out into the open by asking questions. For example: "I get the feeling you assume I'm not telling you the truth; is that right?" This question gives you the opportunity to discuss the fact that you see the person in a different way than she might see herself.

AGREE TO DISAGREE

Agreeing to disagree is an essential strategy when talking about eating problems. Conversations *can* continue even when people disagree. Bringing this up directly can help make difficult conversations go better. You could say:

- "I want to continue talking about these matters, and it's okay with me if we don't agree."
- "How is it for you when we don't agree about these matters?"
- "Can we keep talking even though we don't agree?"
- "It means a lot to me to feel safe enough with you to continue talking about things we don't agree on."
- "I learn from our disagreements. I'd like to keep talking. Is that okay with you?"
- "I want you to know that I respect your views even when I don't agree."
- "I like hearing what you are really thinking, even when I have different ideas."
- "It seems healthy to me that we can agree to disagree and still keep talking; that seems like a sign of our respect for each other."

After a disagreement, it's helpful to remind the person you are arguing with that you're really okay with not agreeing and that you are still there for her.

- "I know we don't agree on diets, but I still like talking to you about these things."
- "You know, I don't think that being thin is the only thing of value, but that doesn't mean I don't want to talk about how we feel about dieting."
- "We agree on some of these matters, but not others. I'm glad we can respect each other's opinions."
- "I appreciate telling you about things that are different from what you think; it means so much to me that we can agree to disagree."

- "Our relationship is strong enough to withstand differences of opinion. That means a lot to me."

Arguing never helps. Once an argument is in progress real communication has shut down, because the only goal of most arguments is to win. If you can stop the conflict quickly and give yourself and the person you care about time to cool down, you'll create a safer environment for difficult talks. Consider that the more you argue your point of view, the more likely the person you are trying to help will want to hold on to his own beliefs.

DON'T LET TEARS THROW YOU

Later on in this book we'll talk about how to handle real emergencies, but there may be other times when the people you care about express their unhappiness. These are special opportunities and we want to get the most out of these times. When someone is upset and emotional they are often more accessible, because their pain may open doors that lectures can't.

First, let the person who is upset know that you can see how difficult things are.

- "What you are telling me sounds so hard. I'm sorry this is so difficult for you."
- "I've read about what you are describing and I can only guess that these problems are different for each person. Can you tell me more about what this is like for you?"
- "I can see that you are having a hard time. You aren't alone. I'm willing to listen."

Don't offer false reassurances or deny that they have a problem. Sitting with a person in pain without trying to fix that pain is a great gift. It conveys that you care and that, no matter what, you are willing to go through the ups and downs of trying to understand another person's unique experience.

LET AN ANGRY PERSON WALK AWAY

If someone exclaims: "I'm done, I can't talk about this anymore!" Don't follow him or keep at him. Don't say, "You won't face your problems!" or "You can't just walk away now!" He will think you are insensitive and feel attacked. He may be worrying that he can't control his temper when he's upset. If you have ever been on the receiving end of this misguided strategy, you know what it feels like to want to leave because you don't feel ready to talk, or you're too angry or think you might say things you will later regret. Recognize that your pushing is apt to lead to a horrible exchange of words that will only make him less willing to talk the next time.

Be gracious. Say, "We can talk about this another time." Or "I'm sorry if I upset you" or "I can see this isn't working, let's try this again later." Conversations always go poorly unless both people want to continue. So, if either person feels that things aren't going well, simply stop. It is even OK to make up an excuse, "I've got to go to the bathroom." Or "I have a headache."

Sometimes it helps to make appointments for important conversations. That way both people can be prepared to handle the emotions and topics they've agreed to discuss.

AVOID USING "SHOULD" AND "MUST" STATEMENTS

You'll be tempted to tell the person you care about what she should do. You may even want to urge her to follow your plan. But none of us takes it very well when someone tries to tell us what to do. Even if someone asks for your advice, offer it as a suggestion. Avoid using the words "should" and "must." These words can make us close our minds as well as our ears. Here are some things you can say instead:

1. **Use "I" statements.** In this way you will be talking about yourself. "I feel scared that you will hurt yourself when I see

you exercising so much." Or, "I feel hurt when you don't call me." These statements are much better than saying, "You must stop overexercising," or "You should call me."

2. **State your preferences rather than making demands.** Say, "I would *prefer* it if we could spend more time together," rather than "You should spend more time with me." Or try, "I *prefer* talking to you when you are calmer," rather than, "Stop yelling at me!"

3. **Ask him to consider an idea rather than arguing your views.** Ask him to consider another way of doing things: "Have you thought about ___?" or "Have you considered ___?" If he argues, you can say, "Just think about it; maybe we can talk more about it later." Instead of saying, "You have to eat with me at least once a week," try "Do you think we could get together once a week?" or "Think about it; I'd love to see you next week."

AVOID GENERALIZATIONS SUCH AS "NEVER" AND "ALWAYS"

It is easy to exaggerate when you are frustrated:

- "You never call!"
- "Your diets always fail!"
- "You're always crabby!"
- "You never do anything but exercise!"

These statements seem to just pop out when we're overwhelmed with someone's behavior. Not only do these statements hurt; they are also very easy to prove wrong. He'll invalidate your argument by pointing out the one instance when he didn't do what you have just said he always does, but by that time it's too late. Since you know you can't unsay it, it's better not to use these words in the first place.

These statements tend to escalate most arguments:

- never
- always
- all the time
- constantly

Instead, give someone the benefit of the doubt. Entertain the possibility that the other person *never* does anything *always*. Say "The last time you told me you'd call, you didn't. What's up?" or "Recently you don't seem interested in going out to eat; do I have that right?"

DON'T GIVE ADVICE UNTIL YOU'RE ASKED: (EVEN IF ASKED—BE CAREFUL)

It's hard to listen to a problem without feeling like you should fix it, but jumping in is not what that person really wants.

> *I was so upset with my husband after telling him about how frustrated I was with gaining all this weight. All he did was tell me how I screwed up my last diet. I just wanted him to listen, not tell me what to do.*

Most of us can identify with this sentiment. The key to handling these situations well is to wait until the person you are worried about has clearly asked you to offer advice or solutions by saying: "What do you think I should do?" Even when someone asks, it's better to ask him what *he* has thought of doing before offering your own ideas.

INSTEAD, TRY USING MINIMAL ENCOURAGERS

It's important for the person struggling with an eating disorder to feel your confidence in her ability to improve. Even when you aren't feeling so confident, it helps to express faith that she will eventually figure out how to manage better. You can do that with brief encouraging comments like these:

- "You'll figure that out."
- "You've handled tough things in the past."
- "You can decide what's best for you."
- "You can do it."
- "I'll see you through this because I know you'll do just fine in time."
- "Give yourself some time; you've got a good head on your shoulders."

Most people actually know what they need to do, they just can't make themselves do it. So reminding them of your faith in their ability to cope is a great gift.

Kindness helps, too. People with eating disorders hear a lot of criticism; critical words are remembered and continue to hurt. Remember that kind words are remembered and can continue to soothe. And that kind gestures are taken to heart. Noting a birthday, an anniversary, a difficult time, or having a thoughtful card arrive for no reason at all, can make a difference.

Part II

TACKLING TOUGH TOPICS:
WHAT TO SAY

Each mind perceives a different beauty.

∞—D AVID H UME

Chapter Five

Talking About Body Image

∞

*T*hose who recover from an eating disorder consistently say that coming to grips with body image and improving self-esteem are what helped them most. Yet each person with an eating disorder has her own unique way of distorting not only what her body looks like, but also what bodies are supposed to look like.

This means that discussing weight and body image will be loaded with the potential for pain and discomfort. And it means that you'll want to keep in mind that each person is unique and complex, so some of the examples in this chapter might fit the person you care about, and some might not.

This chapter describes the body-image distortions that typically occur and the kinds of things that are associated with them: things people might think, things people might do and say. Then it covers ways to talk about these issues in a positive way. These include suggestions for what to say and what to avoid saying, as well as suggestions on how to respond when those with eating disorders talk about their bodies.

ANOREXIA

You will often read that people with anorexia see themselves as fat. It's more accurate to say that most people struggling with this problem see themselves as not thin enough. As long as they can imagine losing more weight, they believe there is more work to be done. When they look around, they want to be *the* thinnest. Not being the thinnest is translated into "I'm too fat."

Many people with anorexia believe that nothing matters other than being thin, and this leads them into a deeper and deeper hole of restricting food and ignoring basic physiological needs. Some vomit to control what they eat; others exercise obsessively, and some simply restrict what they eat. Most use some combination of these techniques. As their bodies enter a starvation mode, they are less likely to feel successful at anything else. Thus their self-esteem is intimately tied to their continued weight loss and the power they have to avoid hunger.

Each person with anorexia has trained his eyes to see any image that isn't skeletal as overweight. Any fat is seen as sinful and unhealthy. Worse yet, as he loses weight, he knows that he doesn't look good. He will usually attribute the uneasiness this causes to being too fat.

According to many sources about two thirds of the people who become anorexic develop this disorder before they are twenty-one. In trying to understand how this disorder takes hold, consider how difficult it is to feel successful and competent when you are a teenager. Young people, who haven't yet figured out how to feel good about themselves, make superficial judgments based on what is assumed to be attractive. They often equate attractiveness with thinness and believe it to be the key to gaining friends, dates, success, and happiness.

Most young people report feeling insecure about their looks. People who develop anorexia usually begin by trying to feel better about themselves by losing some weight. Since losing weight is often met with praise from friends and family, it's not surprising that they then want to secure that approval by dieting more. When they can see no other way of feeling good about themselves, anorexia can become a way of life.

Even though anorexia usually begins during adolescence, some people in their thirties, forties, and even fifties continue to struggle with this problem. Many fear changing and cannot imagine feeling okay about themselves at a higher weight. Others get better as a result of life changes or treatment, but then when they are under severe stress later in life they go back to their patterns of disordered eating and low self-esteem. Those of us who care want to remind them that they have done better facing their feelings at other times and that we are hopeful they will work on their problems without focusing on their weight.

BULIMIA

Often people with bulimia are a normal or slightly above normal weight, yet their self-image is of someone seriously overweight. They believe that horrible consequences will follow from their continuing to weigh what they currently weigh, especially that they will be unlovable or the object of criticism. They assume weight loss is the key to more friends, sexual attractiveness, good self-esteem, and a successful life. Seeing few other options for success, they strive to fulfill all their goals with one strategy—having a "better" body.

People with bulimia often focus on some spot on their bodies that they wish were different. Typically this is the hips or stomach for women, and muscles for men. Since they already see themselves as overweight and unsuccessful, they remain terrified of gaining any more weight and being fat.

Most people who are bulimic wish they could eat more, and feel like failures for not being able to resist food. Unlike people who are anorexic, they don't strive to be skeletal; rather they long to be thin enough never to have to fear eating too much. So they assume, *If I could just be thin I wouldn't have to worry about what I eat.*

Most people with bulimia distort what is normal, like Tim, a nineteen-year-old bodybuilder who was five-six and who longed to be two hundred pounds of solid muscle. He had already ruptured two disks in his back from excessive weight lifting. Tim's father was an alcoholic and unfaithful to his mother, and Tim was highly ambivalent about what it meant to be a strong, competent man. He focused this anxiety on his body and believed that if he could just reach his goal, he would be the man he longed to be.

Seetha saw herself as overweight, even though she had not been overweight since she was in the second grade. Now, at thirty-nine, she was by all standards beautiful. She came from a loving family. She married a man she adored and had three lovely children. For all intents and purposes her life was "perfect." In fact, that was exactly what Seetha expected of herself. She left herself no room for error, and she expected herself to be the perfect mom, the sexy wife, the creative homemaker, the loving friend to those who needed her, and the competent professional at work. She lived in fear that her weight would mushroom to unacceptable levels. She couldn't stop vomiting, because she felt she could not control her binge eating. So she continued to seriously restrict what she ate, binged in the evening, and vomited to compensate. She kept this secret, even from her husband, for twenty years.

Like Tim and Seetha, many people with bulimia blame most of their discomfort and unhappiness on having what they consider an "ugly" body. Or if they see themselves as somewhat okay, it is only because in their minds it's their bulimia that keeps them that way.

Most people with bulimia see themselves as having a weight problem, even when it is clear that they are a normal weight. The problem is that they often see normal weight as a specific number or size of clothing. In reality most of us can be "normal" within a fairly wide range. For most people that means within thirty pounds of an expected number. If the person you are concerned about has no associated health problems and eats a reasonably balanced diet with enough calories to sustain normal activity and some aerobic activity several times a week, her weight is probably normal for her. Remind the person you care about that she has said she wants to have a healthy body and that trying to fit a body mold that isn't hers will only make her unhealthy.

FEAR OF FAT

When it comes to body-image issues, most people don't want to be "fat." That fear drives most eating disorders. People with anorexia fear having any fat; those who suffer with bulimia wish they could have less fat; and those who binge eat fear gaining more fat. We have become a nation obsessed with the dangers of becoming fat. Being able to talk about fat in a reasonable and sensible way can take the sting out of this issue.

We read everywhere that 30 percent of Americans are obese, and some of these people have problems with compulsive overeating and bingeing. As more countries adopt our lifestyle and food choices, they too develop populations with a high proportion of weight problems. In many cultures the ridicule for being overweight is even more intense than in the United States. For example, Japan, many South American cultures, India, and Europe think of being overweight as disgusting and indulgent.

Because fat is seen as ugly, children often express more fear of being fat than of war. Likewise they are more likely to ridicule someone for being overweight than for violence, alcohol abuse, or mental illness. It is almost considered acceptable to be critical of someone else's weight problem because it is seen as a sign of weak moral character and lack of willpower.

It's not surprising, then, in the face of such ostracism, that people who have extra weight feel defensive. They can't walk into a store and buy clothes that fit. They face job discrimination and lower paychecks. Over a lifetime obese women earn 2.3 to 6.1 percent less than their average-weight cohorts. And obese men earn .7 to 3.4 percent less than their peers. As small a disparity as $1.25 per hour less in wages year after year can add up to $100,000 in lost wages over a forty year period. (5.) Overweight people don't see themselves on television except as the brunt of fat jokes. Or they identify with someone like Oprah, who has engaged millions with her war on weight (but not her war on acceptance—despite the fact that her overall health is excellent and she has no acknowledged health problems related to her weight).

In short, people who identify themselves as being overweight are backed into a corner where there is intense discrimination and ridicule aimed at their weight. Regardless of any other achievement or success, people who feel they have extra weight also fear being judged and stereotyped as lazy, self-indulgent, lacking willpower, and having no pride.

Because the obese in our culture have a very critical audience, it's not surprising that many develop eating problems while trying to avoid gaining weight. We are approaching a point of national hysteria over obesity. Paul Campos questions our obsessions with weight reduction in an article in the *New Republic* called "Weighting Game: Why being fat isn't bad for you." He suggests that general lifestyle rather than weight is a better predictor of good overall health, and that the primary problem with obesity may not be obesity, but lack of fitness. There are many overweight and obese people who do not have health problems. He points out that some star athletes would be considered overweight—even obese—using standard BMI (body mass index) recommendations, and that research suggests that dieting and the use of supplements could be "a major cause of the ill health associated with being overweight." So, while our culture criticizes overweight people for not being healthy, the fact is many overweight people may be quite healthy. (6.)

When we talk to people about their fears of being fat we want to encourage them to think about the risks of dieting. They may be familiar with some risks: hunger, light headedness, fatigue. But they may not realize that one of the most important risks of dieting is long term weight gain. And we want them to consider that the pressure to be thin is really a criticism of overweight people for not meeting a standard of beauty celebrated by advertisers because of its ability to sell products. The idea that any fat is bad just isn't true.

Everyone who is healthy has to have fat on their bodies someplace. It's normal, and it is essential for good health. All of us carry some fat (18 to 24 percent for women, and 7 to 20 percent for men). Since people with bulimia are afraid of fat, it's sometimes useful to point out that serious problems can result from having too little fat. In boys and men, low body (below 7 percent) fat can result in mood disturbance and loss of strength and endurance. For women, going below 12 percent body fat can result in missed menstrual periods, weak bones, hormone irregularities, and mood disturbance. (7.) In addition bulimia can cause weakness, dehydration, dizziness, and fatigue as well as tooth decay, chronic bowel and stomach problems, inflammation of the esophagus, and electrolyte imbalances. These health risks are greater than those associated with being overweight.

However, many of you are concerned about people who binge eat and who do, in fact, have health problems related to obesity. He may have diabetes. Or she may have knee, hip, or other joint problems. He may have high blood pressure, may have to take medication, and as a result may have sexual side effects. She may have menstrual irregularities.

He may have chronic back problems. She might have varicose veins that make it difficult for her to stand for long periods of time. He might feel short of breath after walking only a little way. She can't tie her shoes without holding her breath. He is the brunt of jokes and now he is isolating himself. In short, you are concerned because you fear that the person you care about is suffering from problems because of increased weight.

Many people with significant weight to lose have all but given up on their bodies and often distort the social and emotional consequences they endure because they are significantly overweight. They build strong defenses to manage a culture that is cruel to them and justify their situations with rationalization such as, "I like being alone." Or "If he doesn't like all of me, he can't really care about me." Or "Kids are always embarrassed by their parents." Finding ways to reassure someone who is struggling with obesity is essential. Reaffirming your appreciation, commitment, and compassion helps. Here are some things that might help:

- "I hate to see you so full of doubt. I wish there were something I could say that would take that away."
- "I hate to see you so down on yourself; it hurts me to watch you do this."
- "Can we talk about why you don't believe me when I tell you I think you look great?"
- "I like the way you look, and when you tell me that you don't believe me, I feel like you are saying I'm lying."
- "Everyone who is healthy has to have fat on their bodies someplace. I wish you would see that as normal."

Train your eyes to appreciate the full range of sizes and shapes people come in, and take every opportunity to express positive opinions about nontraditional standards of beauty. Since our sense of what is beautiful is generated in a cultural context, it is important to recognize all the influences that shape our views, such as popular culture, media images, and advertising pressures. These things will be the focus of the next chapter.

WHAT CAN WE REASONABLY SAY AND DO ABOUT BODY IMAGE?

Many of us don't realize it, but we frequently refer to body image in the course of ordinary conversation, especially when we meet and greet people and when we catch up with our friends or coworkers. Many of the things we say are so automatic that we don't even think about their implications. Commenting on appearance is part of the polite language we've all learned; it's the small talk we use to break the ice, such as, "You look great. How have you been?" "Great weather we're having—you're looking well." Or "Looks like you've got some sun and lost weight." Or, "She is so much fun and she has such a cute little figure. I miss seeing her." We don't mean anything by it—that's the nature of small talk—but to someone who is struggling with body-image issues these can be heavy words.

What we say can make a difference to people we care about who are struggling with eating disorders. This section focuses on some general ways to deal with body image in conversation. It is divided into three parts: words that hurt, words that help, and responding to what sufferers say.

WORDS THAT HURT

To the person who suffers from an eating disorder, platitudes such as "You're not fat," or "That looks great on you," sound like you don't really "get it." Likewise, "I like a woman who has meat on her bones," or "Throwing up is a nutty way to control your weight." You are talking about something that doesn't match their experience and perspective so you seem out of touch and uncaring. Not the message you want to convey.

Keep in mind that thinking that his body is *not* acceptable is excruciatingly painful. It helps to empathize with that pain while recognizing that you won't be able to change his thinking. If you really don't know what to say, let him know you care by saying, "I can see this is painful for you. I'm so sorry this is hard. I wish I could tell you something that would be helpful." If you really don't know what to say you can change the subject. Most important, if you think you said the wrong thing you can acknowledge it.

Most eating disorders involve several body-image issues. We have divided them up by problem types, but really these problems are interwoven, so reading all the sections will help you understand the whole spectrum. Here are some suggestions for what to avoid.

For people struggling with anorexia, don't say:

"I wish I could catch anorexia for a week—that might help me lose some weight."
People make comments like this in offhanded, jovial ways, but someone who has an eating disorder may either feel diminished or applauded. She could feel diminished because she knows you don't understand the suffering that accompanies an eating disorder. Worse yet, she could feel that being able to resist eating is an admirable state that requires great willpower and that you wish you could do that as well.

"I wish I could lose weight."
Even simple comments about how you wish you could lose a few pounds reinforces for the person suffering from anorexia the assumption that there is nothing more worthy of praise than losing weight. It's better and more thoughtful to keep conversations away from the merits of weight loss.

"You look too thin."
They will hear this as a compliment, not a criticism, and many will feel like it is necessary to lose more weight in order to continue getting these commendations.

"You'd look better if you were a little heavier."
To the person with anorexia, gaining a few more pounds and looking better is a contradiction in terms. It doesn't compute. Plus, just by phrasing it this way, you are implying that she isn't pretty the way she looks now. Rather than making her want to put on weight, this will make her want to lose even more.

For people with bulimia or for those who are overweight, don't say:

"You have such a beautiful face."
To most of us, that's a lovely thing to hear. For the person struggling with a poor body image, it's like the kiss of death. He may have heard

this a million times, and he knows it's a euphemism for what he doesn't have. Many people struggling with these issues will take this as an insult. They may smile through it and thank you, but inside they will feel hurt and betrayed.

"You are really attractive. Do you know how beautiful you'd be if you were thinner?"

You are trying to be encouraging. To point out not only what you see but also the potential of what you see. But what the person struggling with obesity hears is that you are deliberately not looking at the rest of her; yet that is the part of her that really, actually, counts.

"That dress looks lovely."

This is risky territory, and might work well for a husband complimenting his wife (see chapter seven on touch). On the other hand, the person with anorexia or bulimia might be afraid she is filling the dress out too much, and the person with obesity will think to herself "But not like on a size ten"—and feel patronized.

"You look so healthy."

You are trying to say that you think he looks good, has energy, and seems fit. But the person with an eating disorder, even if she is in recovery, may clench inside at what looking healthy might imply about her lack of thinness. The overexerciser will probably take this as encouragement to do more of the same. What he hears is that he is succeeding and people are noticing. To him, this is great regardless of the health risks he is taking.

When the person you care about is obese, whether or not he is healthy, he is apt to feel sensitive to people trying to say something nice or appropriate. He will think you are just trying to avoid a comment on his weight and that you are reaching for something to say because you can't say he looks attractive.

"Doesn't she look great?" or "Doesn't he look toned?"

You may not mean to imply that you are comparing the person you are talking to with the person you are talking about, but that is what she will feel. If she weren't struggling with an eating disorder, she might feel just a little twinge of discomfort and wish you were saying this about her. But if she is struggling with body-image issues, this kind of statement can be very hurtful and even push her further into the disorder.

Comments like these send an unintentional message: how noticeable appearance is and how important it is to you personally. On one level, he may realize it's just a way of making conversation, but on an emotional level he feels it differently. A comment about how good someone else looks can feel like a knife piercing flesh. And it is those feelings that fuel an eating disorder.

For everyone who has body image problems, don't say:

"Wow, you look better."
Most of us would appreciate hearing this if we'd been unwell. For those with an eating disorder, though, it only addresses the outside—the physical being we see—not the inside, which might not be better yet. For some it could suggest they weren't so sick after all, and they could fear the loss of attention and support. To others it could suggest they've gone too far in the direction other people want them to go. Or it signals what they most fear: why? At one time you thought they looked bad. And since you probably never said you thought she looked bad, she will continue to assume that she can't trust what you are saying now.

"Looks like you are making progress."
This phrase seems so innocuous, so positive. It would be appropriate and reinforcing in so many other situations. Here, though, it reinforces the wrong thing. By emphasizing the word "look," it makes someone's appearance the barometer for success—be it health, progress, or improvement. So instead of moving away from body image as a major concern, our very language embraces it.

"Hey, you look happier."
Again, the word "look" is a charged word. It suggests that you judge by appearances, that if the surface looks okay then the whole person—inside and outside—must be okay. And this can put a lot of pressure on someone struggling with an eating disorder. Instead of feeling that yes, she does feel happier, she might sense *your* need for her to be happier, and may let you have that reassurance even if it's not really true.

"You look fine. It's not like you're fat or anything."
You are trying to reassure her that there is no need to restrict, purge, exercise obsessively, or try fad diets. What she is likely to hear is, "Stop having an eating disorder," which will seem way easier said than done.

She will fear disappointing you if she can't stop her disordered eating. When you ask her to accept what she finds unacceptable, she is likely to distrust your ability to understand her true feelings. Also the person with an eating disorder doesn't want to be "okay" in the way she looks. Her image is not the image she wants to see in the mirror. She doesn't want to be seen as average; if she thinks you see her that way, it may only push her to try harder to be seen as special.

"Oh, everybody has some there."

You might be tempted to say this when someone looks in the mirror, grimaces, and grabs her gut. Her very tiny gut. You think it's reasonable and could help. Unfortunately, it's not reassuring. Some people don't want to be like everyone else. To the person who has embraced anorexia, even the teen who wants to fit in and be like her peers in so many other ways, being the skinniest person is what matters most, anything that feels like fat (any flesh that she can pinch) feels disgusting to her.

"Come on, tell me how much you weigh. I'll bet you only weigh a hundred and one."

Coworkers are just making conversation with a little teasing, but meaning it in good fun as gentle humor. They think this will be taken as a form of flattery. For the person trying to recover, for the person trying to build up, this feels like an intrusion into privacy, particularly since those saying it tend to make it a regular conversational gambit. The people saying this may not realize that the person they are talking to might have a disorder, or they don't understand how serious it is. Deflecting comments like this take up a person's energy. And if the person is not in recovery, 101 might sound like too high a number.

"You can gain five pounds in a day. It's normal."

We all experience small fluctuations in weight and take them in stride. For the person who is restricting or purging, though, these fluctuations rule their moods. To them, a few pounds can seem grounds for panic.

Here are some other things to avoid saying:

- "Are you trying to kill yourself with this?"
- "I can't believe you'd do something so stupid."
- "Can't you see how sick you are?"

- "You're making me crazy just thinking about this."
- "You're upsetting everybody with this problem. Get a grip!"
- "You've gained twenty pounds. What's going on?"
- "You're too fat."
- "You look like a boy."
- "You look like you're going to break."
- "You've become an eating machine."

Actions and Words That Help

Many of us assume we are supposed to be critical of our bodies, so we discuss our own dissatisfactions in everyday conversations: "My thighs are so big, yuck," or "I hate my hair," or "I can't believe I've gone up a size; how depressing." This is because our culture doesn't make it seem right to be satisfied with one's body.

This leads us to say and do things that only reinforce negative body image in others. There are a number of small things you can do to change that in your own life. These can make a difference to the people around you who are struggling with eating disorders.

Since eating disorders are linked to body dissatisfaction, the road to recovery is paved with many conversations about body image. Take small steps that promote more positive thinking. Here are some important things you can do:

Stop talking about weight

Take note of how often you criticize your own weight and vow to stop criticizing yourself or anyone else for being overweight. Don't say, "I'm so fat," or "I look terrible," or "If only I could lose ten pounds." Don't talk about your own eating in negative terms, such as, "I ate so much at the party; it was so disgusting," or "I can see that hamburger on my huge thighs." Any reference to fat and being disgusting is a trigger for people with eating disorders to assume you think they are disgusting.

Recognize that every time you criticize your weight—or anyone else's, for that matter—someone around you will wonder what you think of his or her weight. Realize that criticizing your weight is probably a way to get some reassurance that you look okay. Try to validate yourself by reminding yourself that you are okay and that you don't need a "perfect" appearance to get what you want and need.

Be especially careful around young children, because they absorb our self-criticism as an indication that being overweight is the worst possible outcome in life.

It's not enough to stop saying critical things about weight and bodies. It's also important to take the whole subject off the table. It's not helpful to ask people about their diets, or the diet pills they are using, or how they stay so thin. You may be trying to compliment them. You may be trying to connect with them in some way. These kinds of conversations are so ingrained in us that it is easy to continue having them with other people in our lives at the same time as we are being careful not to have them with someone who is struggling with an eating disorder. But these comments can be overheard, and the person you are talking with might have an eating disorder you are not aware of. The underlying message of these diet questions is that you think the person you are talking with looks good and looks thin. People with eating disorders of all ages—from seventeen to seventy-two—report that when important people in their lives tell them how good they look, the more they lock into the importance of continuing their destructive eating habits.

Think about what you admire (other than weight)

Every time you think about complimenting someone for losing weight, think of something else to recognize, such as her kindness, talents, accomplishments, skills, or why you value her friendship. Point out the things that you like about other people. Take every opportunity to give compliments about small acts of kindness. Be sure to say how much and why you enjoy someone's company.

Emphasize what your body can do more than what it looks like

Point out how happy you are to have a body that can ___ (fill in the blank with things like "dance, skate, ski, sing, pick up a toddler"). Talk about what an amazing thing a body is by admiring all the wonderful things it does for us outside of our awareness, like breathing, fixing our wounds, and remembering things. Since our bodies are where we live, celebrate your home.

Throw out clothes that don't fit, and encourage others to do the same.

If you can't bring yourself to throw out clothes that don't fit, at least don't say derogatory things about your body like:

- "I can't wait to fit into that dress."
- "I keep this outfit as an incentive to get thinner."
- "I'd rather not buy anything new if I have to go up a size."

Remind others that keeping or getting clothes that don't fit is an invitation to a bad mood.

- "Giving those jeans away will make you feel better. I gave away my jeans that don't fit as a way to tell myself I'm okay at any size."
- "I like the way that outfit fits you; don't pay attention to the size."

Respect your body's basic needs and take good care of it.

Feed it. Exercise it. Enjoy its versatility. Appreciate its uniqueness.

More specifically, here are some things you might say:

Anything you say about the things that inspire you to feel positive about her without reference to weight or body type will be helpful and appreciated. Take some time to think about the things you notice and value that aren't related to image. Share those thoughts generously. Open your arms and your heart with enthusiasm for the opportunity to spend time together. Say, "I can't wait to see you!" "I love spending time with you," "You're awesome!" and "I love you." We all feel better hearing that those we care about value having time to spend with us.

When thinking about things you can say about body image to people who are struggling with feeling that their body is not acceptable, remember that they already feel less than perfect. You'll want to be generous with praise whenever you can, so point out things you value unrelated to appearance.

"There is so much more to life than being thin. I notice that you are good at . . ."

Talk about their strong points. "You're great at bridge," or "I love the way you arrange flowers," or "I wish I were as good as you are at math." Even when your comments seem to go unnoticed, your positive comments will be appreciated.

"I wish you could see yourself as others see you."

It helps to point out that others are more aware of her strong points than she might be. Making clear that you have heard others praise her successes will help. Pointing out that you know she doesn't see herself as successful but that others do helps to reinforce that the way she evaluates herself is out of line.

"I feel like a failure when I try to be perfect."

Many people who suffer with anorexia see any mistake as a total failure. When people can't allow themselves to make mistakes, they can't learn anything new. When you can talk about how you have learned from your mistakes, you open the door for a kinder approach to the inevitable errors we all make. Start by acknowledging that we all make mistakes. Talk about what dieting has meant to you: "Diets always make me feel like I'm failing because they're so hard to stick to." Then talk about how this has changed for you: "giving up dieting has taught me to value qualities besides my appearance." Keep the conversation going by asking, "What's that like for you?" Let them mull it over. At some later time you could say, "How are you doing with the perfectionism stuff we talked about before?" Talking about perfectionism can be a relief for both of you compared to disagreements about food. And, after all, it may be the perfectionism that is really driving the eating problem.

"I know you like that thin look, but to me it doesn't look so healthy."

When you can acknowledge that she likes how she looks, you let her know you understand her views. But since you don't think being very thin is attractive, you can help by saying that you prefer a fuller figure because it looks healthy to you.

"You're a beautiful person."
When you focus on the whole person, you are letting him know that you are looking past the outside. That what you see is the inside.

"I see such joy in you."
When you speak to the person, not the body, you can help them change the way they view themselves. And when someone's self-image changes, she will feel different! "When my self-image changed I felt different. I felt attractive and beautiful in a way I never had before in my entire life."

People often forget the emotional lives of those who struggle with obesity. They tend to act as if people with obesity don't *have* emotional lives. This is sad. People with obesity have the same deep feelings and strong passions as everyone else. Yet they develop reputations for being jolly, easygoing, placid, with nothing much disturbing the tenor of their days. In effect, they become emotional eunuchs in other people's eyes— and because other people don't want to see it, they don't show their pain.

"You have no idea how much of a help you were on this."
Rather than comment on something you can see, comment on something you can feel: her kindness, her maturity, how much she helps others. Help her realize her self-worth, and help her connect it to who she is, and to the things she does that show the kind of person she is. You don't value her for her looks; remind her of the things that make her special to you.

"I am such a klutz, scatterbrain, or nerd. But you don't see me that way, do you?"
Maybe the person with the eating disorder has teased you about it gently, maybe she has given you a hard time for focusing on it, and maybe she has made a point of pointing out what's neat about you. When you talk about your own foibles, you give her the opportunity to bolster you, and you open the door to a conversation about self-image, and how common it is to see oneself differently from how one's friends and family do. What's important is that this statement doesn't put any pressure on the person to talk about herself or her issues. It is indirect. It shifts the focus of the conversation onto you, the person who does *not* have an eating disorder. Yet in implying all the ways in which the person you care about values you, you are letting her know there are all sorts of ways in which you value her.

If the conversation takes off and shifts back to her, great. If not, no problem. When you say something like this you plant a seed in her mind. Let it sit there and put down roots. If you try to force it, she may toss it away.

"I think I said the wrong thing here, didn't I? It was stupid, right?"
Saying this can defuse a situation. It might also get the person you care about to tell you what would be better to say. (For "stupid," you could substitute "silly," "insensitive," "off base," "ignorant," "wishful thinking," "intrusive", etc.)

Every chance you get, look for openings in conversations. You'll want to encourage those you care about to see the bigger picture and to appreciate the fullness of what it means to be a healthy person. A balanced sense of self often begins by seeing ourselves reflected in others' eyes when they reaffirm the qualities they enjoy in us.

RESPONDING TO WHAT SUFFERERS SAY

People who are preoccupied with weight often need and seek reassurance. It is easy for us to feel exasperated with having to go over the same ground over and over. We get fed up because we wish what we say would take immediate effect. Instead, it helps to realize that repeated conversations on the same themes are the most successful ways to change deeply ingrained fears. Your patience will be easier to maintain when you accept that you'll have these conversations many times and when you have some things to say in response.

"Do I look fat? Do you think I've gained weight? Is my butt too fat?"
The first time you can answer in one of these ways:

- "No, you don't look fat."
- "It isn't."
- "That's not true."
- "Your body is very beautiful and attractive."

The second time you can say, "I told you." The third time you can say, "I'm not going there." The fourth time you can say, "I told you; I'm not going there." Just refuse to participate in the conversation after that. Let her know you're happy to talk about something else.

Sometimes the person you care about will bring up issues of body image himself. He is trying to find out if he is restricting enough, purgeing enough. He might refer to himself; she might compare herself to others. And they might persist in asking the same questions over and over. You don't have to keep on answering those questions; that will only reinforce the thought process.

"She's skinnier than I am, isn't she?" "I'm fatter than she is, aren't I?"

Your first response can be straightforward:

- "She's not a healthy weight."
- "Yes, she's skinnier, but she's not healthy."
- "No, you're not fatter than she is."

Then you may want to follow the same process as above. Or you might want to discuss the way our culture gives us messages about our bodies that can take over our thoughts. The next chapter focuses on how that works and how to talk about it.

"She's prettier than I am." "All the guys at school think she's hot and I'm not."

Just about everyone has thoughts and feelings like this, and one doesn't need to be struggling with an eating disorder to experience it. If you're a parent or a friend, ruefully telling a teenager that you can remember that happening to you is probably not going to help. But you can point out that "You hear about her and she probably hears about you."

Looking at yourself through the media is like looking at one of those rippled mirrors in an amusement park.

∞ —EDMUND S. MUSKIE

Chapter Six

Talking About Messages from the Media

∞

*T*he media bombards us constantly. We look to these sources to inform us about trends in health, fashion, and diet. But we're not just getting facts; we're getting value judgments. Entertainment stars are thinner and more muscular than most of the rest of the population. Fashion and fitness magazines invite us to purchase not only the magazine but also some sort of diet or exercise program. Our mailboxes overflow with unsolicited catalogs tempting us to buy an improved image. Regardless of the body type that is the current fashion, we are told we don't measure up and need to aspire to whatever today's standard of beauty seems to be—that all we have to do is buy in now and we, too, can have it all.

On the plus side, it is often easier to get people to talk about the media than it is to get them to talk about themselves. It's less personal, less threatening. It's easier to have a conversation about what is on TV or what you see in a magazine than to talk about how someone is personally suffering from the effects of an eating disorder. For example, saying something negative about a TV show or a magazine article is easier than confronting someone's bulimia head-on. Likewise, saying how hard it is to feel positive about your own body when you read fashion magazines is easier than saying, "Your body image is way out of line."

BODY IMAGE AND THE MEDIA

You might think that only those with low self-esteem could be manipulated and influenced by the media. But frankly, we are *all* vulnerable to doubt about our bodies. TV, movies, billboards, magazines, and music videos all send the message that a better body will mean a better life, especially in terms of love and sex.

Our young people are particularly vulnerable when bombarded with these images, often computer-enhanced, that try to sell them on the basic belief that they aren't okay. The more they strive to meet the prevailing mainstream image—the look that's in—the more likely women are to value thinness above all other attributes, and men are more likely to value extreme muscularity. Sadly, the more they try to achieve these goals, the more likely they are to develop an eating disorder.

Here are some important facts compiled by the National Eating Disorders Association: (www.nationaleatingdisorders.org) (8.):

- 81 percent of ten-year-olds are afraid of being fat.
- The average American woman is five-four and 140 pounds. The average American model is five-eleven and 117 pounds.
- Most fashion models are thinner than 98 percent of American women.
- A majority of Caucasian middle school girls read at least one fashion magazine regularly.
- Most of these magazines contain an article that highlights how weight loss improves appearance.
- These magazines also highlight stories about the primary value of exercise being "to become more attractive" and "burn calories."
- A study of 4,294 network television commercials reveals that one out of every four commercials sends some sort of "attractiveness message," meaning they tell viewers what is or isn't attractive. That means adolescents see on average 5,260 "attractiveness" commercials per year.

Regardless of ethnic background and culture, young people are over-whelmed by messages about how they are supposed to look and by the call to diet, have an extreme makeover, wear "in-style" clothes, do rigor-ous exercise, and keep buying things that will bring them closer to a standard that no one really fits. We need to be prepared to talk about these images and their impact not only on them but also on ourselves.

Teens plaster these pictures inside their lockers and on their mirrors to remind themselves that they aren't okay and that they need to im-prove. Women in their thirties and forties often believe that once their weight falls outside "the zone" their appeal is gone forever. For men there is a double whammy, because not only do men's health magazines portray lean images, they also suggest that "the healthy man" needs to be incredibly fit and muscular.

We need to challenge these assumptions and ask ourselves:

- "Why do I buy these magazines?"
- "If I don't fit the images I'm looking at, how do they make me feel about myself?"
- "Would these exercises really work?"
- "Would there be any point in buying these products?"

And we want to make sure that we have people hear us talk about these struggles. Think out loud within earshot of the person with the eating problem.

- "It's too bad we criticize ourselves for not looking like celebri-ties, especially when they don't even look like the pictures of themselves."
- "Real women actually have to have fat on their bodies, and real women *are* healthy and beautiful."
- "I think I need to retrain my eyes. The media has done a real job of convincing me that fat is ugly, but this simply isn't true."
- "I feel better when I look at real women instead of fashion mod-els. How do you feel when you look at these superslim models?"
- "These images upset me because they are so unlike the real peo-ple I know and love."

- "It's great to see someone willing to have herself photographed as she really is." (See the Resources section for reference to an actress who did this.) (9.)

EXAMINING BODY-IMAGE MESSAGES IN THE MEDIA

Conversations about the media are generally not threatening even to those who have severe eating problems. Actually they have the potential to be lively and interesting. It's not hard to raise interesting questions that make people think (and we provide some examples at the end of this chapter). The media are trying to change our thinking and actions. We can turn that around if we pay attention and realize that we can *choose* how to think about ourselves when we:

- see advertising images of thin, "beautiful" people as a way to make us feel bad enough about ourselves so that we will buy what they're selling.
- acknowledge that these images are artificial constructions, often enhanced by a computer, to remove all blemishes, wrinkles, and folds of fat.
- remember that we see only what the advertisers want us to see.
- are clear that we have choices. *We* can choose to look to other sources to compare ourselves.
- learn to criticize the messages we see in advertising. Put sticky notes on them to express what we don't like.
- tear out the pages in magazines that make us feel bad and see how many are left.
- consider not buying magazines that contribute to making those we care about feel bad.
- talk about how what we see in fashion or fitness magazines makes us feel.
- establish lists of companies that consistently send negative messages about people who are not thin.
- notice how all diversity is obliterated in advertising: People of color look like Caucasians, and all models have the same slim hips, ski-jump noses, full lips, and widely spaced eyes.

Examining Diet Messages in the Media

The best-seller lists are full of diet books, and it's hard to find a magazine that doesn't contain an article about weight loss. It makes it seem as if there is something conceited about not thinking we should lose some weight. We feel guilty when we eat certain foods, and wonder about the merits of one diet plan over another.

The pictures of celebrities on their covers beckon us to turn to them for advice on dieting, and so we do. Yet every book and magazine offers contradictory advice on how to eat. Without going into the drawbacks of various diet plans, we should always question:

1. losing more than two pounds a week. Only very overweight people will lose more than that without losing muscle, which is counterproductive. Dehydration, the major cause of more severe weight loss, is dangerous.
2. promises of quick weight loss, which are only a long-range plan for regaining even more weight. 95 percent of people regain all the weight lost within a year, plus additional weight.
3. why someone five-eleven needs to weigh 125 pounds. Realize that keeping weight low for women of childbearing ages increases their risks of having a low-birth-weight baby, which is a cause of developmental delays.
4. the value and the cost of prepackaged meals (some plans cost several hundred dollars a week).

WHAT CAN WE SAY?

The previous chapter focused on how detrimental it can be for people to think that their bodies define who they are, and on how important it is for us to reinforce the things that really matter—the things that make up the whole person. However, there are times when you might want to initiate a discussion about bodies seen in the media. The key is to talk about it theoretically and not in terms of how the person you care about fits any particular profile or type. Let her draw her own conclusions.

Here are some things you might say to raise awareness about how the media influence our body image:

"What a makeup job!"

That puts the emphasis on the artistry rather than an actor's or model's actual physical attributes. It suggests that what you are seeing is contrived, not real. And it opens the door to discussing the image as probably being different from what the real person is underneath.

"I wonder what she really looks like."

This can lead to a discussion of photo angles, photo retouching, digital enhancements, and other technological approaches to altering a person's appearance on film. And to the question of why one would aim for a look that doesn't even exist.

"They make it look as if thin is all there is!"

Remember to say this as an observation about the media, not about someone with an eating disorder. If she doesn't say anything in response, drop it. Let the phrase reverberate in her mind. If she does respond to it, there are all kinds of places the conversation can go, such as talking about:

- the people who are hurt because they think they don't measure up.
- the people who are hurt because they lose confidence in themselves, think they won't be successful socially or in careers, and no longer aim for the same things.
- the people who end up hurting themselves in their effort to change what they look like.
- how standards of beauty vary over time and in different places.
- what body types are really like in the real world and where thin fits in.

"Everyone who is healthy has to have fat on their bodies someplace. What they are showing isn't normal!"

It's great to have an opening to talk about this, because fat cells are not just unavoidable; they're a necessity. Fat is part of people's diets and part of the body's makeup. There are body processes designed to break down fat and there are body processes designed to make use of fat. The body needs fat as it needs muscle and blood cells and organs and glands. Fat helps to regulate body temperature and is a source of energy. When it falls too low, it affects menstruation and the ability to conceive a child. Too little of it, and we become more susceptible to disease. There should be no value attached to fat. It is the word for a substance we need to survive—just like protein, carbohydrate, mineral, and vitamin.

"First they make it seem that everyone has to look like that. And then they sell us all kinds of stuff so we can fool ourselves into thinking we can look like that."

Talking about the profit motive shifts the conversation away from the person with the eating disorder. It suggests we are thinking and acting under someone else's direction rather than as a result of our own conscious choices. It can make us think about where our money goes and who benefits.

"They make it look easy—relaxed, happy, and thin."

That's the trap so many people fall into. It looks so easy for models and actors and wrestlers and bodybuilders. Someone with an eating disorder can't understand why it's so easy for people in the media to look so good when it's not easy for him. They may not realize how false it really is—the specially designed clothing, cosmetics, and photographic technology. For many dancers, wrestlers, models, or jockeys the effort is not just complicated but unhealthy, even potentially life-threatening. And just as expensive in terms of time, money, and the people, things, and activities that are given up.

"Maybe there's such a thing as too much muscle."

This is a way to spark a discussion about what people find attractive and how much that differs from one person to the next. Some people find a lot of muscle disgusting because it's out of proportion or intimidating. You can also talk about "being too skinny" and how that doesn't seem appealing. The point to stress is that standards of beauty change, and some aren't so healthy, such as binding feet, stretching necks, or going to extremes to gain muscle or lose fat.

At the bottom of things, most people want to be understood and appreciated.

Chapter Seven

Talking About Touch

∞

We convey our feelings for each other by the ways we touch. A pat on the back, a hand held, a kiss, an embrace all have meaning. Usually these gestures convey our affection and enhance our connections. On the other hand, many who are self-conscious about their bodies feel worried when we approach.

- Evan avoided all gestures of affection. A hug only reminded him that he was "skinny." He was convinced that every time Tanesha put her arms around him, she was wishing she were with someone more muscular.
- Janis saw herself as fat, despite being a normal weight. She avoided intimate situations because she assumed the rolls she felt on her waist would also disgust those close to her.
- Brooke wanted to be open to her boyfriend's touch, but she couldn't be because she was preoccupied with her weight. She found it impossible to allow any physical contact because she didn't want to be criticized for being too thin. Her boyfriend broke up with her because he didn't want a girlfriend whom he couldn't touch.

People with eating disorders are torn. They long to feel accepted and valued, yet they often feel unworthy of affection. Your willingness to demonstrate your affection with touch, despite the difficulties, has the potential to deepen your relationships and strengthen your bonds. Even more important is your willingness to talk about touch, because those conversations have the potential of easing some of the conflict.

Here are some things you can do and say.

TALK ABOUT TOUCH

For people with eating disorders, touch can be threatening even when there is nothing romantic or sexual about the relationship. At the most basic level, touch means coming into contact with flesh. To the person with an eating disorder, who is not comfortable with her own body, or not proud of it, touch can reveal what she perceives as grave deficiencies. She may find her flesh disgusting to her own touch and shudder when she anticipates the revulsion someone else might feel on touching her. Though part of him may miss the warmth, comfort, and affection expressed through touch, if he is struggling with anorexia or obesity the risk may not seem worth it.

Most people with body-image issues, and that is most people with eating disorders, worry about touch. They fear that every time someone touches them, they will feel disgusted. A romantic or sexual connotation compounds the problem. The person with an eating disorder is convinced that she is not attractive even to look at. When someone touches her she becomes more intensely aware of her own body and how it feels at the place that's being touched. So it is not only the revulsion of the person who touches her that she dreads; she can't stand to feel that touch herself.

Touch is very important to relationships, particularly romantic ones. And it is very painful for the other person in the relationship to lose the comfort, the nourishment, the intimacy, and the bonding that touch brings. Talking about it can be difficult. If you are that other person in the relationship, you can become hurt, frustrated, and insecure. This, in addition to the eating disorder itself, can put a real strain on your relationship. It's important to let the person you care about know that it feels good to touch him and why, by saying things such as:

- "I love the feel of your skin."
- "It makes me happy just to put my arm around you."
- "Holding your hand makes me feel special."
- "It makes me sad that you don't see how wonderful it is to be close to you."

MAKE SURE YOU HAVE PERMISSION TO TOUCH

Ask before you touch. We like to think that affectionate gestures arise out of the spontaneous affection that two people feel for each other and are always welcome. But unfortunately, that isn't always the case. To be on the safe side, you can ask questions like:

- "Can I give you a hug?"
- "Is it all right if I put my arm around you?"
- "Can I touch you here?"

If you notice that the person you want to touch seems uncomfortable, ask if your perceptions are true.

- "You seem uncomfortable when I ___. Are you?"
- "I don't want to make you uncomfortable. Am I?"
- "Can we talk about what makes you uncomfortable?"

FOCUS ON ENJOYING TOUCH

An important antidote to feeling self-conscious about one's body is to pay more attention to what a body can do rather than what it looks like. That requires shifting focus to the pleasurable feelings that are experienced when you touch and are touched by people you care about. Talking about that pleasure is reassuring but also threatening. Make sure you are clear that you will stop whenever she's uncomfortable and that you won't push for more. Then remind yourself not to push. Tell her how good she makes you feel. Let her know that you also want to contribute to *her* feeling good. It's okay to point out that when she re-coils and seems scared of you, you feel rejected. But this is also a good time to let her know you understand why she is pushing you away and that you'll try not to take it personally.

BE SENSITIVE TO HOW WEIGHT SHIFTS CAN CHANGE RELATIONSHIPS

For example, Maura had been heavy most of her life. As an overweight teenager, she had enjoyed the confidences of her male friends. She accepted invitations for activities late at night and never questioned their intentions. She felt safe. When she lost a lot of weight, men suddenly wanted more than just conversation and advice about how to handle their love lives. They were interested in a sexual relationship with her. She was lost and didn't know what to do. She had no experience, but because she was an adult, people assumed she did. So men sometimes complained that she had led them on, and women friends criticized her for being naive.

On the other hand, Sean had always been attractive to women and grew up with many more opportunities to date than he could handle. But when he became overweight as an adult, women were no longer interested in his sexual advances. He assumed he was doing something wrong, but didn't consider that his weight was a factor.

As the friend, family member, or partner, it's hard to know how to help the person you care about figure this out. Try to be positive and affirming by expressing your confidence that she can handle these changes. Sympathize with his upset and confusion and consider saying, "It must be really hard to understand why you are getting these reactions. What do you think is going on?"

TALK ABOUT SEXUAL ATTRACTION

It is not unusual for couples to have trouble talking about how weight affects their sexual feelings. And it's normal to be afraid that our sexual feelings won't be reciprocated. Most of us can relate to this fear, which makes talking about sexual attraction difficult. And because it is so difficult, most people avoid this topic whenever possible. People who fear that their weight is unattractive withdraw and are often afraid of saying or doing anything that will bring on the rejection they fear. The people who care about them are often afraid to say anything because they don't want to make matters any worse. That leaves no one talking and everyone fearful.

It's important to know what to say. So here are answers to three common questions. Keep in mind that these are just suggestions. Your own intuition about what to say and what not to say should be your primary guide.

Should I talk about my feelings of attraction?

You know that your sexual feelings are influenced by his appearance. You also know that you want to avoid being hurtful. That creates a dilemma. Say something and you risk hurting the person you care about. Say nothing, and you risk continuing to withdraw, which also damages the relationship. If the relationship is important to you and you care about maintaining strong sexual feelings, yes, risk saying something. If you don't care that much and you know you will be hurtful, you might just as well avoid causing pain.

Usually people don't want a real answer to the question, "Does my weight make me unattractive to you?" They want reassurance. Even if they don't ask the question outright, it doesn't mean they aren't harboring fears that you and other people will find them unattractive as a sexual partner. Almost anything you say about attraction can't be unsaid. To the person who is suffering, a "yes" will feel like pressure to change immediately, which, of course, isn't possible, and so it will feel frustrating.

Nevertheless, if you are in a marriage or a long-term committed relationship that is suffering from lack of sexual connection, you'll need to figure out how to address this sensitive issue carefully. If you aren't sure how, you might talk with a mental health professional skilled in these matters.

If you *are* attracted to the person you care about, be generous with your reassurance. Provide all the evidence you can to make your attraction and interest clear; take every opportunity to reaffirm your feelings and commitment. And be patient, because most of these conversations need to happen multiple times.

Will it motivate him to lose weight if I tell him I'm no longer attracted to him?

No, it won't. More than likely he is already worried about how his weight is affecting you, and that awareness has not been sufficiently motivating to change his behavior. Rather than asking you directly, many people who have gained weight express this worry indirectly with comments like, "Wow, I've really gained weight; I hope you will still love me." This is a window of opportunity for you to reaffirm your affection while supporting efforts to change with comments like, "I know you worry about my attraction to you, but it is more important to worry about your health. Can we focus on taking better care of you?" You want to redirect their concern to positive things that can be done to make their health better.

Should I tell her she's too thin and that I find her unattractive?

It is often less offensive to be told you are too thin than that you are too fat. And, of course, some even believe you can never be too thin. It is usually safe to say something such as, "I thought you looked better a little heavier," or "I love you, but I'd love even more of you if there were more of you," or "You look healthier with more weight, and I would find that even more attractive."

Words That Hurt

It is easy for words about touch and intimacy to be misunderstood. One of the most damaging things about these misunderstandings is that the person whose feelings are hurt is apt to say nothing at all. This makes it hard for you to get the signals to back off or to say something else. Here are some things to avoid saying.

"I just love your cute big butt." Or "I love those curves!"

Guys may be trying to let gals know how attractive they are finding them, but this is a big turnoff. It doesn't just focus on appearance; it plays into the disgust people can have for their own bodies, and for what they imagine their flesh will feel like to anyone who touches it.

"I love the way you've rounded out."

You want to convey how appealing you find her. But all she hears is that she must have a lot of fat everywhere and that it's obvious to everyone.

"I can't wait to touch you all over."

You're letting him know how sexually attractive you find him. But it triggers his fear that you are going to find out how very unattractive he really is.

WORDS THAT HELP

Having the perfect thing to say is not important. What is important is that she hears how much you care about the relationship. Try to be relaxed, open and warm when you bring the subject up. Focus on asking rather than telling. Let her take the lead. If the conversation seems too tense, just say how much you care and would like to understand, and then back off.

"Tell me where I can touch you. Tell me when."

This puts the power back in the hands of the person with the eating disorder. If she doesn't know where and when the touch is coming, she will be on guard and may cringe. If, though, you let her tell you, she can feel prepared and more comfortable about it. It may be that there are certain areas of her body that are off-limits (often the stomach), or maybe she can't tolerate your touching her bare skin. If you can work these things out, she will gradually become more accustomed to touch and, in a romantic relationship, begin to feel she is attractive.

"It helps me so much when you touch me. I would like to express the same to you."

When you say this, you help her think about touch in a different way. Touch is a way people show caring. It needn't be much—a touch on the shoulder, a pat on the hand, an arm about the waist, a ruffling of hair. What's important to understand is that it's love flowing out of someone's hands, that it's not so much about touching a body as it is about touching a person. And that's what you want—each of you expressing love to the other.

"This is important to our relationship. Let's see if we can figure out a way to make it work."

Ask for his help. Be satisfied with small things at first. It's a lot harder than it looks, but it is possible to build up slowly. Don't put on a lot of pressure. Don't make him feel shamed or ridiculed for having difficulty with touch. In his situation, it takes a huge amount of trust to allow any touching at all. If he's thinking about any kind of touch, he is already taking huge steps forward.

Talk it over. Never act first; ask first. Be ready to accept that one time might be yes and another time might be no, and that someone might take one step forward and two steps back. If the only way she can consider being touched is while all covered up, let that be, too. Any kind of touch is a starting place. And let her set the pace, because pressure will only set you back.

"Touching is part of communicating in this family. I don't think I can give it up altogether. Just tell me where's okay."

In many families, touch is a language in itself. And in families where words aren't dominant, touch can be glue that binds people together and a lubricant that eases tensions. Messages are passed back and forth without words. People touch to say hello and good-bye, to let someone know that everything is okay, to show agreement, to show they care, to ask a question, to remind someone of something, and any number of other things. Without touch, the whole communication system can break down, and people can begin to feel more and more isolated from the person they love who has an eating disorder. You can bring the subject up. You can suggest there be some new rules about how touching can work.

"It always feels so good to touch you."

She may not believe this at first. If she had a weight problem, people might have commented on softness or flab. If she was anorexic, people might have commented on her bones. Even if what was said was intended to spur someone to get treatment, it's hard to forget hurtful comments such as; "You feel like a bag of bones," or "You look like a boy." With statements like that dancing around in her head, not to mention her own sense of disgust at her body, it can be a long road toward feeling okay about touch.

But it is important to keep telling her that she is attractive, especially if she is in recovery and struggling with body-image issues. She has to feel there is an upside to what she is doing. If she is working hard to make progress with an eating disorder, she needs you to be more supportive and affectionate. You might say:

- "You have a sparkle in your eye instead of that dazed look."
- "Your hair looks so nice and shiny."
- "You look pretty today."
- "That's a cute outfit."
- "I can see a difference in your eyes, like you're here with me."
- "You make my heart sing."

"I love touching your stomach, resting my head in your lap."

Let her know that you love that she is comfortable as well as attractive and that you enjoy being with her, doing things with her, eating with her. This is the person you care about; you like the whole package, inside and out. Tell her that.

"I love being able to get close to you again."

When you say this to the person who has been restricting and couldn't bear to be touched, it has a strong emotional component, because physical intimacy isn't the only thing you will both have missed.

For people who struggle with obesity, there is also a physical reality to this statement. As people gain significant amounts of weight, sex can become difficult. The obese person can even lose physical touch with his own body and feel disengaged from it. As he starts to lose weight, sensations start coming back. Even at the simplest level this weight loss can make a difference. He will be able to reach certain body parts again—just getting dressed, bathing, tying shoes will become much more doable. And touching another person becomes physically easier, too. Instead of being difficult, maybe impossible, requiring a lot of compromises, sex can become more mutual, more sensual, and more fun. That one's partner feels all these positives, too, is both rewarding and uplifting for the person who has been battling obesity successfully.

"Did you hear the joke about the . . . ?"

How you touch a person's mind and heart is important, too. There are ways we talk about touch that clearly imply sexual intimacy. We use jokes, innuendo, sidelong glances, flirting, and tone of voice. When we do this, we are letting people know that we see them as sexual beings—that this is part of their wholeness and their humanity. People who struggle with obesity often find that they are no longer included in conversations of this sort. Women, particularly, feel stripped of their sexuality and sexually invisible—it's not just that others don't find them interesting that way, but that it's almost as if it's assumed they wouldn't have any interest in sex themselves.

He who fights against monsters should see to it that he does not become a monster in the process.

∞—FRIEDRICH NIETZSCHE

Chapter Eight

Talking About Diet—Avoiding
Food Fights

∞

*W*e generally assume that what someone else eats is really none of our business. We might invite a friend to go for a pizza, or a child to come along for an ice-cream cone, but we don't demand they eat all the pepperoni or only half of the ice-cream cone. Essentially, we don't pay much attention to what someone else eats. But when we sense a problem with eating, many of us go on high alert, and it feels wrong to say nothing. This chapter talks about how to handle these feelings and what to say and to avoid.

It's hard not to notice when someone is eating in a way that seems destructive.

1. Will eats over 3,000 calories a day, most of it after five P.M. He begins the day promising himself that he'll do better, so he skips breakfast and then grabs a Power Bar for lunch. By dinnertime he's famished, and so eats second helpings of everything. Later in the evening he rewards himself for having "been good" all day by eating ice cream, chips, and cookies.

2. Tasha always tries to keep herself below 500 calories a day. A typical day of eating consists of a breakfast of strawberries with Cool Whip Lite (90 calories), a lunch of lettuce and baby carrots with fat-free dressing and a soft pretzel (185 calories), a snack of three corn chips and five Gushers

(65 calories), a dinner of nine mini rice cakes and a dessert of candy hearts for 210 calories. If her daily count goes over 500 calories, she will punish herself the next day by allowing herself nothing but water.

3. Katie feels that on a "good" day she eats "healthy." For her, "healthy" means no carbs and no fats. So that leaves her eating meat, a few fruits, and nuts. She eats egg whites for breakfast, sliced turkey for lunch and dinner. She will allow herself a piece of fruit daily and a handful of nuts sometimes. When this routine breaks down and she eats "forbidden foods," she forces herself to vomit.

One of the toughest things for friends and family to negotiate is how to talk about food. It's tricky to know whether to comment, when to comment, how to comment. Do you push people to eat because they need to gain or discourage them from eating when they are bingeing? Do you tiptoe around mealtimes, lock up food, sneak around and spy on them, only feed them what they want, constantly make food available?

Here are some of the common questions that come up about food and eating, and some suggestions for what you can say and do.

WHAT IS NORMAL EATING?

While there is really no one right way of eating for everybody, Ellyn Satter, MS, RD, LCSW, BCD, provides guidelines for normal eating in her book *How to Get Your Kid to Eat . . . but Not Too Much.* (10.)

Normal eating is being able to eat when you are hungry and continue eating until you are satisfied. It is being able to choose food you like and eat it and truly get enough of it—not just stop eating because you think you should. Normal eating is being able to use some moderate constraint in your food selection to get the right food, but *not* being so restrictive that you miss out on pleasurable foods. Normal eating is giving yourself permission to eat sometimes because you are happy, sad or bored, or just because it feels good. Normal eating is three meals a day, most of the time, but it can also be choosing to munch along. It is leaving some cookies on the plate because you know you can have some again tomorrow, or it is eating more now because they taste so wonderful when they are fresh. Normal eating is overeating at times: feeling stuffed and uncomfortable. It is also undereating at times and wishing you had more. Normal eating is trusting your body to make up for your mistakes in eating. Normal eating takes up some of your time and attention, but keeps its place as only one important area of your life.

In short, normal eating is flexible. It varies in response to your emotions, your schedule, your hunger, and your proximity to food.

People with eating disorders may not realize that restricting what they eat can boomerang. Restricting often leads people to indulge in forbidden food or greater amounts of food, and then the indulging leads to even stricter restricting. And this can become a tortuous, painful, and self-destructive pattern.

Sometimes, showing empathy for this vicious cycle can bring people who suffer to question—in their own minds—why they are doing something that entraps them this way. Sometimes, getting into a theoretical conversation about what people think normal eating is can accomplish the same thing. This is because the conversation is not about this particular person, but about the various ways people might define normal eating. What both these approaches have in common is that they don't attack the person and her eating habits. This is important. Pushing for change can reinforce her defenses for the path she is on.

You could open a discussion by saying, "With all this information about diets, it's hard to know what's normal. What do you think?" Or you could ask, "What do you think normal eating is?" If they ask for your opinion, you can offer some of the characteristics listed above.

Should I tell someone else what to eat?

Generally speaking, it's a bad idea to try to convince someone to eat in the same way you do or in some way that you think would be healthier. If you do, two problems occur: First, you'll miss the opportunity to say, "If you're concerned about how to eat maybe you should talk to a professional. Would you be willing to consider this option?" And even worse, you set the stage for her to lie to you to hide what she is actually doing. When that happens you can't talk about what is going on. Most important, monitoring someone else's eating means trying to control what you cannot control, and that will only make you feel out-of-control and irritable.

But there are many things you can say that might help, such as:

- "I can see you are really struggling with what to do about this problem. I'm sorry this is so hard."
- "Trying to not eat what you want to eat seems like torture. Is there anything I can do that will help?"

What if he asks, "Do you think I'm going to gain weight because I let myself eat that?"

Regardless of the eating disorder, one item isn't going to make a big difference to weight in either direction. Just say so. If the person is restricting, you could say, "I can't imagine that it could." If the person is struggling with binge eating, you could say, "I don't see how one could hurt," and you might add, "It's stopping at one that's always hard for me."

Should I confront someone who is eating too much (bingeing)?

The answer to this question depends on whether or not they have asked you to intervene when you see them eating too much. And even when someone asks you to step into this role, you might want to consider saying:

- "I really don't want to be in the role of telling you to stop eating when you seem to want to eat. If I do this, I risk your being angry with me, especially if you want to continue eating. And I care about you and I care about our relationship, so I don't want to be your food monitor."

When you watch someone eat too much who clearly has a problem, it's hard to say nothing. But sometimes you must honor the fact that people have a right to decide what they eat. You can say something like:

• "I'm worried about the choices you are making about food, and about how our relationship might be affected if I talk about how you eat."

What should I say about dieting?

We live in a dieting culture. In fact, chatter about the merits of one diet over another occupies considerable amounts of conversation time, probably second only to the weather. There is evidence that girls as young as nine or ten feel better about themselves when they are on a diet. One survey of college women found that 91 percent had attempted to control their weight by dieting. We know that about 25 percent of American men and 45 percent of American women are on a diet on any given day. (11.) So most people—and that includes us—have feelings and ideas about diets.

We also know that 20 to 25 percent of all dieters will go on to develop eating problems. (11.) In fact, most eating disorders begin when someone attempts to lose weight by dieting. Some experts even believe that dieting is responsible for most eating problems. Here are some compelling facts that are worth repeating:

• Most diets don't work. Ninety-eight percent of dieters regain their weight within five years, and 90 percent of those gain back more weight than they lost. (12.)
• If you don't eat enough to maintain your body, your body begins to consume itself. Most believe they are losing fat; yet study after study shows that dieting destroys muscle, bone, and even brain tissue.

- Dropping below 1,400 calories a day for most adults will result in losing tissue that is not fat.
- The Framingham study, published in the *New England Journal of Medicine* in 1991, found that dying from a heart attack is more likely in those whose weight fluctuates (yo-yo dieting) than in those whose weight remains stable, regardless of their initial weight, blood pressure, smoking habits, cholesterol level, or level of physical activity. (13.)
- High blood pressure can be a side effect of the mental and physical stress of dieting.
- Low levels of potassium and dehydration (an electrolyte imbalance) put a severe strain on your heart.
- Studies find a direct link between dieting and osteoporosis. This disease leaches calcium from the bones and results in significant bone loss.
- Dropping below 15 percent body fat causes menstruation to stop, which results in estrogen-deficiency illnesses and infertility. It is also believed that the act of losing weight by itself is enough to stop menstruation in some women, even when they do not drop below 15 percent body fat.
- The list of illnesses associated with dieting is long and includes: anxiety, depression, lethargy, lowered self-esteem, decreased attention span, weakness, high blood pressure, hair loss, gallbladder disease, gallstones, heart disease, ulcers, constipation, anemia, dry skin, skin rashes, dizziness, reduced sex drive, menstrual irregularities, amenorrhea, gout, infertility, kidney stones, numbness in the legs, reduced resistance to infection, lowered exercise tolerance, electrolyte imbalance, bone loss, and osteoporosis.
- The end result of most diets is weight *gain*, which precipitates another attempt at dieting, which leads to temporary loss followed by weight gain. This is often referred to as yo-yo dieting.

If someone you care about isn't overweight but goes on a diet anyway, you'll probably be concerned. Ask her why she wants to lose weight, what she thinks this diet will do for her. If she says, as many do,

"I just want to feel better about myself," it might help to ask why she doesn't feel good about herself as she is.

- "It doesn't seem to me that your weight is a problem, but I hear what you are saying about wanting to feel better about yourself. What else besides your weight do you wish you could change?"

It also helps to say that you do not think she has a weight problem and to invite her to consider whether other issues are making her feel bad about herself.

- "I don't think your weight is a problem; what's up with that? I don't get it."
- "There is so much evidence that diets don't work, and you seem to be a normal weight. I'm confused why this seems like a good idea to you."
- "I don't think your weight is the problem. Do you think something else might be?"

You can also point out that when someone who doesn't have a weight problem talks about losing weight, it makes others who do have a weight problem feel terrible. So when Susan says, "I have got to diet," Claire, who is heavier, suffers and worries that Susan thinks she is fat. Help people see that when they talk about diets around others who see themselves as heavier, they have the potential to hurt them.

What should I say about the holidays? I'm worried about all the eating that goes on at Thanksgiving and other celebrations.

Holiday meals are difficult, and people with eating disorders can dread them for weeks ahead of time. It means dealing with temptation. It means seeing people one doesn't see often who are likely to comment on one's appearance. Concerns about weight and appearance can be so much on their minds that they may say they want to skip holiday gatherings altogether.

Acknowledge that family gatherings are stressful for most people. Since we don't get to pick our families, it might help to acknowledge the challenge of being with people you didn't choose. You might even say, "I'm not very excited about this holiday either." If you're in the same family or will be attending the same event, try saying, "I was really looking forward to your company/spending time with you," to show that you care about enjoying the time to reconnect, and that you aren't concerned about who is eating what and who has gained or lost weight. Take the focus off the food and refocus on the fun. And if fun is not a realistic alternative, focus on just getting through the day.

What about people who are seriously overweight? How can I talk to them about dieting?

Generally we want to encourage people to be healthy, and losing weight is often a healthful step. It is fine to support positive efforts in that direction.

However, most of us get frustrated when people don't follow through or when they aren't able to take our advice. Then our relationships can suffer. Because the dieter worries about disappointing us, it's a good idea to avoid giving specific advice in the first place.

Instead, when people who are overweight and in medical danger tell you they want to try this or that diet, offer general support. Don't chime in with opinions. You might say:

- "I can see you really want to feel better. That's great."
- "I want to support you. How can I help?"

This makes it possible to be a source of support through all the ups and downs.

What can I say when the diet he plans to try seems silly?

Support the effort without supporting the diet plan. Many people who struggle with their weight try one plan after another. Unfortunately, we can often see that what they are currently trying is apt to fail because the program isn't balanced and doesn't include lifestyle changes that include eating less and exercising more. You'll want to avoid the "I told you so" attitude. Rather, help him see that it is really "dieting" that is the failure, not him as a person; it's not that he doesn't have enough willpower.

If he is ready to try something else, suggest consulting a dietician who has experience working with people making lifestyle changes that can lead to sustained weight loss. What he sees as a failure is really an opportunity to try something else that might work. Let him know you see it that way.

What should I say when she doesn't eat enough?

When the person you care about doesn't seem to be eating enough, try to talk about what you have observed without sounding judgmental.

It's tricky because the person you care about may adopt several strategies. She might eat more to make you think things are okay and then vomit or overexercise to compensate. She might take more food but push it around the plate, feed it to the dog, or spit it out into a napkin. Pushing him to eat more could make him feel like he is disappointing you if he doesn't think he can make those changes. Instead, it might be more effective to say:

- "I notice how often you criticize yourself for eating. It hurts me to see you holding back on foods you used to like. This seems to be causing you trouble—what do you think?"

What should I say when she insists some foods are good and some are bad?

Many people with eating disorders identify certain foods as good (usually vegetables and fruits), and others as bad (usually fats or carbs). Don't get into heated debates about what constitutes correct thinking about food. Don't suggest a diet plan that you have found successful.

Instead talk about food as "fuel" and "necessary nourishment." Remind them that all foods are okay in moderation. Remind them that when we restrict certain foods, we almost always develop cravings, and cravings make us feel like failures when we give in.

Sometimes it is useful to talk about emotional eating. We all have comfort foods that we like to eat when we are anxious or upset, typically foods that are high in fat or sugar. When people you care about seem to be using food for consolation, you might want to suggest that there might be better ways to satisfy their basic needs. Again this might be a time to point out that professionals are trained to help people identify what they need and how to best satisfy those desires.

What should I do if he wants me to help him with his diet?

Helping someone count his fat grams and carbs is not a good idea; nor is agreeing to diet together. There are several problems with involving yourself in someone else's diet plans. First of all, he may be hoping you'll supply the motivation he doesn't feel. When that fails, he may end up disappointed in you. Second, these well-meaning gestures create a competitive environment where the focus is on winning. So it's usually best to simply say:

- "I don't want us to compete. I want us both to feel successful."
- "I think you can handle that part (or this diet) just fine. What else could I do to be supportive?"
- "Losing weight is a real challenge. I'm glad to talk about how I've struggled, but I don't want either of us to feel bad about not succeeding."

Should I talk about portion sizes?

Yes and no. It's not a good idea to point out that someone is about to eat too much. For example, you don't want to say, "I can't believe you are going to eat that whole thing," or "That's too much." On the other hand, in a more general way you can talk about how portion sizes have grown and that many of us have trouble figuring out what is a reasonable amount to eat on any one occasion. There is even some interesting research showing that as a nation we are eating larger portions. For example, Samara Joy Nielsen and co-author Barry Popkin, both professors of nutrition at the University of North Carolina, found some interesting results using data from national government surveys of food consumption taken between 1977 and 1998, and the time period during which the proportion of Americans considered obese grew from 14.5 to 30.9%.

- The average size of a hamburger grew from 5.7 to 7 ounces which adds on 97 calories

- French fry portions increased from 3.1 to 3.6 ounces adding 68 cal
- Soft drink sizes roses from 13.1 to 19.9 ounces increasing calories by 49
- Among people under age 39, pizza and salty snack consumption rose as much as 143 percent (14.)

What should I say about supplements?

In the United States, drug manufacturers are required to prove that drugs are safe and have met rigorous screening before being sold to the general public. However, under the 1994 Dietary Supplement Health and Education Act (DSHEA), the FDA can remove a dietary supplement only after it has already been marketed to consumers and that *then* has been proven unsafe.

Consumer Reports listed these six substances as definitely hazardous or very likely hazardous with the following explanations (15.):

- Aristolochic acid (aristolochia, birthwort, snakeroot, snakeweed, sangree root, sangrel, serpentary, serpentaria, Asarum canadense, wild ginger)
  - Dangers—potent human carcinogen, kidney failure, sometimes requiring transplant; deaths reported.
  - FDA warning to consumers and industry about an import alert; in April 2001 banned in seven European countries and Egypt, Japan, and Venezuela.
- Comfrey (Symphytum officinale, ass ear, black root, blackwort, bruisewort, sonsolidae radix, consound, gum plant, healing herb, knitback, knitbone, salsify, slippery root, symphytum radix, wallwort)
  - Dangers—abnormal liver function or damage, often irreversible; death reported.
  - FDA advised industry to remove from market in July 2001.
- Androstenedione (4-androstene-3, 17-dione, andro, androstene)
  - Dangers—increased cancer risk, decrease in HDL cholesterol.
  - FDA warned twenty-three companies to stop manufacturing, marketing, and distributing in March 2004. Banned by athletic associations.

- Chaparral (Larrea divaricata, creosote bush, greasewood, heniondilla, jarilla, larreastat)
  - Dangers—abnormal liver function or damage, often irreversible; deaths reported.
  - FDA warning to consumers in December 1992.
- Germander (Teucrium chamaedrys, wall germander, wild germander)
  - Dangers—abnormal liver function or damage, often irreversible; deaths reported.
  - Banned in France and Germany.
- Kava (Piper methysticum, ava, awa, gea, gi, intoxicating pepper, kao, kavain, kawapfeffer, kew, long pepper, malohu, maluk, meruk, milik, rauschpfeffer, sakau, tonga, wurzelstock, yagona, yangona)
  - Dangers—abnormal liver function or damage, often irreversible; deaths reported.
  - FDA warning to consumers in March 2002. Banned in Canada, Germany, Singapore, South Africa, and Switzerland.

It's important to realize that you can't control what another person does with these products, but you can at least express your concern and refer them to these three Web sites that contain reliable information on herbs and supplements.

- The National Institutes of Health at http://www.nih.gov/
- Memorial Sloan-Kettering Cancer Center at www.mskcc.org/mskcc/html/11570.cfm
- ConsumerReports.org

What if she goes to the bathroom after eating and I know she is planning to vomit?

Please consider saying nothing. She knows what she is doing is not a good idea. Most people who have bulimia only get more upset and more secretive when they feel people are watching what they are doing. When she goes to the bathroom after eating is not the right time to say something, because she is already overwhelmed by the urge to vomit.

However, you may want to say something at another time, when she is calmer and open to a conversation about her eating problem. You might ask about how she is doing with this, and even more important, you might ask how she feels about the fact that you notice and that you are concerned about what she is doing to herself.

- "You told me about the problems you are having with bulimia; is it okay to ask how that's going?"
- "Do you mind my asking about how things are going with the eating problems you talked about?"
- "I noticed that you go to the bathroom after you eat. Is it okay to ask about that?"

But shouldn't I try to stop her?

No, you shouldn't. The end result of most attempts to stop bulimics from vomiting is that relationships fall apart. It is sad for people who are already struggling with an eating problem to also worry that friends and family are so disapproving that they'd try to force them to stop vomiting.

Averil put it this way: "My roommate won't talk to me anymore. At first she seemed concerned when I told her I was bulimic. But she just expected me to stop vomiting right away. I couldn't. And now she won't talk to me. If I were an alcoholic she might have given me more time to work this out. But no, she didn't, and now I've lost her friendship."

On the other hand, Tyrone had this experience: "My family knows I'm struggling, and it really helps to be with them, because they don't follow me to the bathroom and try to stop me. But I want them to think I'm doing better, so when I'm with them I try to not vomit. I don't feel nervous and that helps me relax, eat normally, and then do something else besides vomit."

What if the bulimia is creating a biohazard?

Some people who suffer with bulimia are not sensitive to the fact that others are left to clean up their messes. Adrienne insisted on vomiting standing up, and so left vomitus all over the floor and sides of bathroom stalls in her residence hall. The resident director was worried that confronting this problem would only make the bulimia worse. But not confronting it left other residents angry and did nothing to help Adrienne be responsible for herself and her behavior. It is reasonable and necessary to insist that vomit be cleaned up and sanitized.

Some people who have bulimia vomit in plastic bags and leave it in places that create biohazards. It is reasonable to point out to those who create these conditions in shared spaces that this behavior is not acceptable. Just be straightforward about it. You're not telling them to stop being bulimic; you're just asking them to keep things hygienically safe for everyone.

- "I'm worried about you, and I'm sorry this problem is so difficult for you. But we need to make sure that you are not creating problems for others. Can you agree to clean up after yourself?"
- "If you want to get help to stop vomiting, I'd be happy to give you some leads, but in any case, please make sure to clean up after yourself."
- "I know it's not your fault that you have this problem, but like the rest of us you *are* responsible for any mess you make."

Reaffirm your caring and concern and follow up several days later to see how it's going.

What about the studies that show people live longer when they are really thin?

You may have heard about the CRAN diet (Calorie Restricted Adequate Nutrition) and the claim that severely restricting calories can increase longevity. In animal studies the animals that are kept very thin do, in fact, live longer. However, what we aren't told is how these animals behave. They are irritable, aggressive, and will frantically search for food when given opportunity. They act like creatures obsessed with getting food.

Thomas Wadden, director of the Weight and Eating Disorders Program at the University of Pennsylvania, says the classic study on calorie restriction, involving twenty healthy young men who cut their food intake in half for six months, found many negative effects, including "marked signs of depression and irritability." The subjects "were despondent, had very low energy and had lost the initiative to do things. They began to hoard food, and when allowed to eat again, they indulged in binge eating." (16.)

What could you say to someone thinking about this plan? You might say to someone who is trying to justify severely restricting calories:

- "I can understand wanting to live longer, but you seem so irritable since you started this plan. Do you notice a difference?"
- "It seems like there are trade-offs, maybe some positive outcomes, but also some negatives. Are you okay with that?"
- "I wish you would think more about how your moods are altered when you don't eat well."

SOME GENERAL DOS AND DON'TS

Here are some general dos and don'ts to keep in mind. The rest of this chapter will suggest things to say and not to say and explain why.

DOS	DON'TS
Encourage family meals.	Don't make food a reward or punishment.
Be supportive of reasonable attempts to manage diet.	Don't talk about yourself as being "good" or "bad" related to what you have eaten, such as, "I was good today; I didn't eat too much."
Encourage good intentions.	Don't talk about your weight struggles and your desire to resist certain foods, or how bad you feel about your own weight.

DOS	DON'TS
Encourage three meals a day and moderate snacks.	Don't try to limit a child's caloric intake—unless requested by a physician for medical problems.
Encourage enjoyment in meals and conversations. Keep it fun. Laugh a lot.	Don't push or force anyone to eat or not eat.

There is only one constant: Take the focus off food. Don't constantly make it part of conversation; don't roll your eyes or use other body language to show that you're watching and judging. Here are some things to avoid saying as well as some ideas to approach conversations about food in a positive way.

WORDS THAT HURT

"You are going to eat this." Or "Eat this now." Or "I won't let you do this until you eat that."

This makes food a fight rather than an enjoyment. It's demeaning as well as threatening. People with eating disorders already have negative feelings about food. This only adds to them by making sharing meals a negative thing, too. Many people will just tune you out if you say this.

"You are not going to eat that, are you?" Or "I think you've had enough."

Pushing someone *not* to eat is as bad as pushing someone to eat more. It puts the spotlight on eating, on the disorder, and on the person with the disorder. It takes away from the time you are spending together and suggests that this is all the relationship is about anymore. Ironically, in trying to promote healthy eating you are creating an unhealthy situation.

"You haven't eaten all day." Or "I haven't seen you eat anything."

You say this because you care and because you want them to know you are trying to watch out for them. What they hear is that you are spying on them. They will feel cornered and resentful. If you say this in front of others, they could feel isolated, embarrassed, and even humiliated. The last thing they'll want to do is comply. It would make them feel submissive and in a childlike role.

"Can't you eat just a little more—for me?"

You are hoping a little nudging will help. That maybe he'll eat out of love and respect for you, or because you need so much for him to do so. But all he hears is pressure. That his efforts just aren't good enough. That you are disappointed in him. He may have put forth a tremendous effort to eat at all. He's done the best he could, and now all he wants is to run from the table. When one's effort is never good enough, it's easy to stop trying.

"I don't understand why you can't eat one little ___."

When someone is restricting, this just adds to the pressure. You might be trying to express your frustration, or hoping she will open up and tell you why this is so difficult for her. But she doesn't know how to explain it. And even though she understands that you don't understand, part of her hears you saying that this shouldn't be so hard and that all it should take is a little willpower. That is both wounding and demoralizing. And it can make someone feel that you no longer respect her. Since self-esteem is a big part of eating disorders, this can make her struggle even more difficult.

"I don't understand how you can starve yourself to death . . . (or stuff yourself to death)."

He doesn't understand it either. But saying it doesn't help. It feels intrusive, and it can feel like an attack. To some, it can feel as if you are saying they are crazy. Also, this is one of the things that people with eating disorders hear often. They don't have an answer for it. If they are not ready to get help, it's not going to inspire them to do so. If they are getting help, it suggests they are not making progress. Either way, it implies that they are making bad choices and that you think they can change. So saying this can feel like an attempt to make them feel guilty. That doesn't help the recovery process.

"Can't you see what you are doing to yourself?"

You may say this with anguish. You hope that awareness will prompt him to get help. But this feels intrusive, too. It can feel as if you think he is stupid. Or he may feel that yes, he does know what he is doing, and he is doing it because he wants to. Either way, it is unlikely to prompt the kind of productive conversation you are hoping for.

"This is just food. How can you have a problem with that?"

You say this because you are struggling to understand where they are coming from, and it looks like it's all about food, but often it is not about the food per se. It's food through which people are expressing feelings, hiding from feelings, trying to build self-esteem, trying to control something else. Once someone becomes entangled in an eating disorder, it is not so simple to stop.

It can take years of therapy, effort, recovery periods, and relapses. Even though they are not addicted to food, the struggle, the obsession, the traps, the pull of it, the demands of mind and body, can be similar to what someone suffering from an addiction experiences. It can be hard for friends and family to look at food this way. Food is so normal, ordinary, healthy, bodybuilding. This doesn't fit with what we know, with what we have experienced. People don't need drugs and alcohol to live, but we do have to eat. So the dynamics are different. It's not a black-or-white situation where someone can say this is something he will eliminate from his life forever and avoid ever being near so as not to be tempted by it. Because of the differences, many people with eating disorders hate being labeled "addicted" and dislike analogies that compare their eating problems to a drug or alcohol problem. They want you to know that having an eating disorder is hard to overcome, just like an addiction. But it's not the same for two reasons. First, food is not a mind-altering substance, even though it can be used for comfort instead of nourishment. And second, you can't give up eating without serious health consequences.

"You must promise to tell me whenever you feel like doing this."

It's one thing to offer to be a backup, or to be the person someone can go to when she doesn't think she can stop herself from satisfying an urge. It's another thing to insist on being a backup. It doesn't help to insist. And in this case it can feel like one step down from spyware or a wiretap. You can't demand to be joined at the hip.

"Hey, you finally ate something." Or "Wow, you ate so healthy tonight."

Of course you mean well and you're trying to be supportive, but this still puts too much emphasis on food and makes people feel they are being monitored. It's not for you to comment; it is for them to bring it up. If they comment on their success, great! Then you can respond. But avoid saying, "I noticed." Instead, tell them how glad you are for them. You can simply say, "Hey, that's great."

It's important to keep in mind that when you say something along the lines of "Oh my God, you're eating!" it can make the person who is restricting want to stop eating.

"You didn't eat enough." Or "Aren't you eating too much?"

The first will make the person with anorexia recalculate calories. The second will make the binge eater feel resentful and guilty. Both can make the person with bulimia ready to purge.

You are trying to be helpful, but the person you care about will hear something else: that you think you know exactly what he needs and are trying to tell him that. As hard as it is to keep silent, we have to bite our tongues. If you think about it, you probably don't like unsolicited advice or other people assessing you, either.

"How can you not eat that when it looks so good?"

Ironically, to the person with anorexia, this sounds like a compliment. It can make her feel good because it says that she has control. So saying this to entice her to eat only reinforces not eating.

And saying this to someone struggling with obesity or compulsive eating doesn't help either. Especially in restaurants and at holiday meals, people who are trying to eat healthy are bombarded with comments like this. And those who are saying it don't usually stop with just one comment. They say it several different ways, apply a lot of pressure, say

"What could it hurt?" or "Just try a couple of bites," or "You have to have something," or "You're really missing out here," or "This is one of the best things I've ever tasted." Even the waitstaff can get in on the act: "Look at all the choices," or "Try it; it's our specialty." And their body language suggests it's crazy not to. To the person who is trying to eat differently, this isn't a onetime thing. It's tantamount to falling off the wagon and could make it all the harder to stay with the program the next day, too. Sadly, even if they manage to resist at the restaurant, this can set up such a craving that it can catch up with bingers and compulsive eaters once they get home.

This can be an issue at the workplace, too. People will bring leftovers from a meeting or reception and urge others to go and partake. They will say things such as, "Don't forget to go down and get something," or "You can use it," or "I brought something in just for you." They think they are being kind and helpful. Or they may be teasing a little: "Is that salad enough for you?" or "Saving for a big meal tonight?" Sometimes meetings will take place over drinks or over meals. This makes it difficult to control the kind of food and the amount of it. It's somehow understood that the meeting won't go as well if everyone doesn't participate in the eating and drinking. That makes for a lot of pressure.

"I really shouldn't be eating this, should I?"

Even though you're talking about yourself, you are making food the subject of the conversation, suggesting there's an issue involved, and making her the authority on it. Move the conversation somewhere else.

"Don't you get hungry?" Or "Aren't you starving?"

Maybe you are trying to encourage someone with anorexia to eat. Maybe you are trying to commiserate with someone who is trying to eat healthy and control obesity or bingeing. But it's irritating to the person who hears it—partly because so many people will say this; partly because neither wants to think about the hunger he is feeling.

"You eat the same thing every day. Don't you want something else?"

For people with eating disorders, setting up a system simplifies things. It helps with focus and it helps with follow-through. It helps with getting food down and it helps with resisting temptation. Any kind of experimentation can derail their effort, so they are very careful about making changes. And this is especially true for people in recovery.

You may just be making conversation, but they hear a challenge to what they are eating. This makes it even more difficult for someone with anorexia to eat what she has committed herself to eating, and it makes it more difficult for someone who is trying not to overeat to stick to the portion controls she has put in place.

Also, for the person struggling with bulimia, it removes an element of safety. She may have figured out what she can manage to eat on a regular basis without a need to throw up or to run several miles to burn it off. You think of it as just eating—and maybe enjoying—a meal. She thinks of it as a chore. It's her task to sit and keep her mind off what she is eating. To not focus on how it feels in her stomach. To live with the feeling of food in her stomach making her uncomfortable. And to not add to what she is eating because that would help her throw up.

"Let's go get dinner."

That sounds so unthreatening. Unfortunately, it isn't. To the person who is anorexic, it is too focused on the food aspects of dinner, and warning bells will clang. To the person struggling with obesity, there's the fear that there will be food that will be too hard to resist, or food that isn't healthy.

Here are some other things to avoid saying:

"How often do you throw up?"
"Why don't you eat something normal?"
"You must have been really hungry."
"Are you sure you want to eat that?"

And don't make comments to someone else about another person's eating habits, such as "Well, she never eats anything." It's not just inappropriate to talk about someone as if she isn't there, it's demeaning. And it can make a person feel invaded and insulted as well as invisible.

WORDS THAT HELP

"Let's get a pizza while we read."

With a person suffering from anorexia, you want to take the focus off the food and not make a production out of it. Instead, incorporate it into another activity. Some variations could be: "Let's order in and watch a movie." "Hey, let's talk about that project over lunch." Or "We'd better grab some breakfast before we go to class." Now it's not a matter of taking time out to eat but of associating the meal with other things. That makes it social—hanging out with friends, something to do while studying. It's easier for someone with anorexia to eat under those conditions. Just keep the suggestion casual.

And if they say, "No," let it go. If you don't, it's not casual and tangential anymore. Just say, "Okay," or "Maybe later." Otherwise it could feel like a con, as if it really was all about eating after all, or even a bit of a bribe or blackmail. The key is to be sincere, not to single out the problem, and to keep the focus away from food.

So often food is the centerpiece of social events. You can help by not making eating the main event. Instead of restaurant meals, set up pool parties, bowling, a bike ride, a walk to explore a neighborhood—all events where food may be involved but is not the point of the outing. And if someone with an eating disorder plans a dinner, respect his plans. Bring only the kind of food you were assigned. Bring only the quantity you were assigned. That shows you care about him and respect his decisions.

"I'm really concerned about you, but I'm not going to force you or treat you as a child. However, I am always going to ask you whether or not you've eaten. I know you don't like it, but that's just how I am."

This is okay because you are being up-front about it. You are asking that he take you as you are and committing to taking him as he is, too.

"Is this the kind of thing where there are triggers? Is that something I could help you with?"

The person you care about might not want to share her triggers. Respect that. If she does share them, just make a note of them. Try not to react with horror, ridicule, or disbelief. Be as matter-of-fact about them as possible.

For the person struggling with compulsive eating, triggers could include something as straightforward as sitting down, or a certain time of day; sometimes they can be associated with certain activities, such as reading or watching television. Certain foods can be triggers, too, like the old potato-chip commercial—"Bet you can't eat just one." Leaving a serving dish out family style could be much harder to deal with than serving individual portions.

Though there are some common triggers, every person will have his own list. This is true for those suffering from anorexia and bulimia, too. For the person with anorexia, some possible triggers are comments about food, being angry or sad, or any kind of comparison to someone else.

If you know what the triggers are you can help to avoid them (if the person you've talked to wants you to assist). Just be careful not to draw attention to them in front of others.

"Are there any things that are the opposite of triggers, such as places that are safe?"

If the person you care about is comfortable about discussing triggers, this would be worth asking, too. There may be places that people never eat (such as the bathtub or the backyard) and places where someone is more comfortable about eating (such as in a particular room or with a particular person). Depending on a person's goals, type of eating disorder, and preferences, you could help by joining him in environments that work.

"How's the struggle going?" Or "How are you doing?"

Talking constantly about the eating disorder is intrusive and can feel patronizing or controlling. But never referring to it isn't a good idea either. It's one of those elephants in the room that everyone can feel. If you go far to the other extreme and say nothing, the person you care about could feel abandoned, could feel she is being judged, or could wonder why you are ignoring this so completely. If he has talked to you about it at some point, asking how it is going is appropriate. If he hasn't, just asking about things in general will show you care. Either way, he can open up and talk as much as he wants, or simply give the easy answers of "I'm fine" or "Thanks for asking." What is important is that you showed you cared, gave him the opportunity to ask for support, and maybe made him feel comfortable about talking to you in the future.

"What do you want to do tonight?"

Talking about going out for the evening demonstrates that here is one relationship that can still feel good and "normal." And that interacting with you is safe—not focused on food or diet or appearance or his behavior, not about trying to make him change.

One of the reasons this message is positive is that people with eating disorders are hoping to hear that people want to spend time with them. Leaving the door open for activities that don't involve food lets both of you enjoy each other's company without having to deal with the temptations of eating situations.

I find the great thing in this world is not so much where we stand, as in what direction we are moving.

—OLIVER WENDELL HOLMES

Chapter Nine

Talking About Exercise

∽

*T*here is such a thing as too much of a good thing. When exercise becomes the focal point of life, when it replaces food or must be done to earn food or erase food, when nothing else—not sleep, not special occasions, not other people's needs—can interfere with it, when it is exempt from any of the occasional shifting of priorities life has all of us make, then it may no longer be a positive force in someone's life.

Most people with eating disorders have a problem with exercise, getting either too much or not enough. Many people with anorexia exercise way too much and are literally running on empty. Those who struggle with bulimia also sometimes overexercise as a way to compensate for what they are eating. This is often followed by periods of not being able to exercise much at all. Overexercising is a typical pattern for men, who often use exercise as their primary source of "purging." Many women use this strategy as well. On the other end of the spectrum, people who binge eat and have gained weight often wish they could get themselves to exercise more.

When talking to someone you think should exercise more or less, keep in mind that they are likely to see your concern as criticism. This chapter will talk about how you can broach the subject without sounding critical or judgmental.

TALKING TO SOMEONE WHO
EXERCISES TOO LITTLE

She knows she should exercise and has reasons why she doesn't think she can. She already feels pressured to do what she isn't doing. So insisting on change won't work. Instead suggest everyday activities that encourage more movement but that don't seem like exercise. For example:

- Take the stairs instead of the elevator.
- Go for a walk during a work break or recess.
- Park the car far enough away so that walking is necessary.
- Blame the dog; remind the person you care about that Fido needs a walk.
- Walk slowly and take breaks so the person you care about feels comfortable walking with you.

Encourage walking. It's good for the heart and lungs; it's a weight-bearing activity, which staves off osteoporosis; and it is the exercise least likely to cause injury. Your invitations are more likely to be accepted when you are able to graciously accept rejection without taking it personally.

If someone complains of stress, lack of energy, sleep problems, or stiffness, remind them of the benefits of exercise:

- Less risk of heart disease
- Less likely to develop high blood pressure
- Less risk of osteoporosis (weak bones)
- Less risk of diabetes
- Less risk of obesity
- Easier to maintain weight
- Increased flexibility
- Stronger tendons
- Less stress and anxiety
- More energy
- Increased endurance
- Less sleep disturbance

- Better memory and concentration
- Less depression

She might say, "I don't have any energy," or "I can't sleep well anymore." You can help out by saying, "It seems a little strange to me, but I realize I have more energy if I take time to exercise just a little. Do you think that would work for you?" Or "I've read that a little exercise seems to help people sleep better. I'm not sleeping so well myself; maybe we should try walking together. What do you think?"

Stick to "I" statements and to talking about what works for you. That will always sound less critical. And ask how the other person feels about what you're saying. Be as direct as "What do you think about what I'm saying?" or "Can you tell me how this conversation is going for you?" or "I'm not sure where this conversation is going." Give them the opportunity to explain what they think.

Avoid arguing. It's easy to get caught up in a battle when every suggestion you make leads to excuses such as, "Yes, but I can't do that because . . ." If that happens just back off and wait for another opportunity. You can say, "It seems like exercising creates more problems for you than it might solve. That's a hard spot to be in."

Is It Safe to Just Start Exercising?

Generally speaking, if the person you care about is under age thirty-five and is in good health it is most likely safe to start exercising without seeing a physician. Otherwise it's a good idea to get an okay as well as some advice from a health care professional about what might be the best way to begin, particularly if there is any evidence of (17, 18.):

- high blood pressure
- heart trouble
- family history of early stroke or heart attack
- frequent dizzy spells
- extreme breathlessness after mild exertion
- arthritis or other bone problems
- severe muscular, ligament, or tendon problems
- other known or suspected disease.

The key is to pick a program that is enjoyable and then to do it slowly. If the person you care about wants some company and is interested in what you do regularly, ask if she would like to come along. Remember to tell her that you aren't doing this for competition and that you would like her with you for the company. Be sure to mention that the old adage "no pain, no gain" is a ridiculous way to think about enjoying anything.

TALKING TO SOMEONE WHO EXERCISES TOO MUCH

Overexercising puts our bodies in a state of depletion and stress. Too much exercise without adequate fuel can lead to feeling exhausted and drained. Muscle aches and fatigue are a sign that someone has exercised too much without proper fuel or recovery time. When this happens muscles break down, and injuries and illness are the likely result.

It can be scary to see someone you care about do something that has a great likelihood of causing harm. Aaron kept running even though he had a stress fracture in his left foot. Jayne, who was a hundred pounds overweight, decided to train for a marathon without talking to her doctor. Evie exercised three hours each day and seemed exhausted most of the time. All of these examples would cause most of us to worry.

If you feel your relationship is close enough and your concern is significant, tell him that you are worried. "I can't help but see that you seem really worn out." "I worry about you. Most of your free time goes into exercising, but you don't seem to be getting much benefit." "I notice that you seem tired and irritable when you are with me." "Sometimes it seem you're in a lot of pain."

If you are the parent of a minor child, you are entitled to set some clear limits. It's okay to say, "I can't allow you to keep running track if you are no longer menstruating, because you are too thin. Continuing to exercise like this will create a health risk I'm not willing to see you take." (More about this in chapter twelve.)

Check back with them. You can say "I know I've told you how worried I am. I'm wondering how my talking about this affects you and our relationship," or "I hope I'm not being too much of a pest here, but I'm worried."

But if he says something like, "I plan to do this my own way. I'm sure it's okay," it is all right for you to reemphasize that your relationship is strong enough to agree to disagree. "I understand you think this is okay, but I want you to know that I'm still worried. I don't want to make you angry, but I'm concerned about your health. Is it okay if I continue to check in with what you are doing?"

What Constitutes Fitness?

Someone who is fit is strong enough to manage recurring everyday tasks, flexible enough to avoid injury during regular routines, and able to endure the basic physical demands of everyday activity. Being fit allows us to live up to our potential by giving us the energy to function well and do what we value. Being fit allows us to feel confident in an emergency, to bear up under difficult circumstances, to deal with stress, to go the extra distance necessary under adverse circumstances. Because having a strong and fit body also influences mental functioning, being fit contributes to being mentally alert and emotionally stable.

Being physically fit involves four basic components: cardiorespiratory endurance, muscular strength, muscular endurance, and flexibility. All of these components are enhanced by a regular moderate exercise regimen. However, someone recovering from an eating disorder may need to restrict exercising until he is strong enough to handle regular routines without injury.

What Is a Reasonable Workout Schedule?

This depends on what the person you care about is trying to accomplish. An Olympic athlete obviously needs a different training schedule than someone trying to maintain overall fitness for general health. Most of us realize that what a thirty-year-old can do easily, an eighty-year-old might struggle with. Likewise when someone is recovering from an illness or eating disorder it's likely that their exercise routines will also need to be adjusted. A reasonable exercise program should include cardiovascular endurance, strength training, and flexibility enhancement.

For most adults a minimum guideline might include a warm-up period where the activity to be practiced is done in a gentle fashion for five to ten minutes, followed by cardiovascular training for at least twenty minutes three times per week. Good cardio activities include brisk walking, running, swimming, cycling, rowing, cross-country skiing, and games like racquetball and handball. This routine would be enhanced by also stretching for at least ten minutes a day. Certainly, more exercise is appropriate for young people or those training for athletic events.

The heart rate most people should maintain during cardiovascular exercise is (220–age) × .70. So a forty-year-old would want to maintain a heart rate of 126.

These guidelines are a suggested baseline for good health. Keep in mind that we can't demand that someone, even ourselves, stick to these standards.

CAN WELL-TRAINED ATHLETES DEVELOP EATING DISORDERS?

Yes. Athletes are at high risk for eating disorders because they often diet in order to meet weight requirements for various events. Since dieting is the leading cause of eating disorders, it's not surprising that many highly trained athletes develop eating problems. And even when there are no weight requirements for a sport, many athletes feel they need a body that is different from the one they have in order to be competitive. This desire can lead them to risky dieting and exercise regimens that are dangerous to overall health.

Female athletes are vulnerable to three fundamental problems called the athletic triad: the drive for thinness, dieting, and amenorrhea. Without their even realizing what is happening, these problems can snowball into other dangerous problems such as osteoporosis, eating disorders, and gynecological problems. For male athletes the temptation to use dangerous supplements, to overuse various muscle groups, to restrict eating, or to overeat in an attempt to gain weight often leads to lifelong complications. Problems such as infertility, joint degeneration, body-image distortions, eating problems, and metabolism disruption that lead to long-term weight gain are not uncommon. And because athletes hang out with other athletes much of the time, this team culture of unhealthy habits can be inadvertently reinforced by teammates, coaches, and others.

If we care about an athlete's health and not just her ability to win, it's important that we risk saying something about the destructive patterns we notice. Our perspective is important, because she may be caught up in an athletic culture where the basic needs for reasonable health are sacrificed. You may know or have read about athletes who:

- exercise six to seven hours a day while also restricting what they eat
- vomit to meet weight limits for wrestling
- Develop depression and exhaustion from overexercising without adequate rest and food-fuel
- embark on fad diets or strict eating regimens
- wanted to quit but who believed their parents, coaches, and friends would be disappointed if they "gave up"
- were afraid the muscles they were developing would make them unattractive
- were afraid of not being big enough or strong enough and so risked taking dangerous supplements

Common sense matters. When someone is engulfed in a culture that is sabotaging his basic health, the voice of reason can make a difference.

So speak up with courage and say what you think. But when you do, also realize that it's important to check out the effect of your comments. You can say, "I'm worried about how my concern is affecting how you feel about me. Please realize that no matter what, I'm here for you. I just hate to see you hurting yourself."

WHAT CAN WE SAY?

Here are some things you might want to avoid saying and some things that could help.

WORDS TO AVOID

"That girl must work out a lot to have a body like that."

Instead of feeling admiration, the person with an eating disorder will immediately apply this to herself. If she has anorexia, she will think, *I exercise a lot and I don't look like that.* If she struggles with obesity, she will think, *I'll never look like that. My body must look disgusting to the person who is speaking.*

Don't comment on anyone's appearance. It can spur some people to overdo it. It can make other people give up.

"Exercise is the best way to go."

Suggesting that to someone who is already overdoing it will make her want to exercise even more. She will hear that she is not getting enough results. It's a general comment, not even about weight, but to someone struggling with obesity, this will seem too simplistic an answer. Maybe trying this in the past hasn't helped. Maybe he's so out of shape that he can't imagine even getting started. Basically this will feel like criticism.

"You look tired and worn out. Why don't you take a break?"

You're trying to encourage some rest and relaxation, but you've really expressed that she doesn't look so good. She is already too concerned about her appearance, so these comments will only reinforce her fears that she is not looking good enough.

WORDS THAT HELP

"It's okay to miss a workout every once in a while." Or *"It's okay to skip a day."*

It's particularly helpful if a weight trainer or coach says this. It adds credibility. No one is perfect. Others don't expect it of themselves or the people around them, so those suffering with an eating disorder shouldn't expect it of themselves either. Let them know it's okay to relax once in a while. The world won't come to an end. They need to give themselves permission to be human.

"Would you like to have a walking/workout partner? That would be great for me."

This can help the person who is overdoing it as well as the person who is having trouble gearing up to exercise or to do it consistently.

For the person who is overdoing it, having you participate helps to put a frame around the exercise and set boundaries in terms of how much and for how long.

For the person who is not getting enough, having a date with you will help make it happen. It can add pleasure to an activity that is difficult or take away embarrassment about exercising in public.

For those not used to going to gyms and fitness centers, it can actually help a lot to have someone to go with, especially for men. Men struggling with obesity don't stay away from gyms just to avoid comparing themselves to people who are more muscular; they may also avoid going because it's assumed that men know how to use all the equipment. They dread asking for instructions, exposing their ignorance, and coming across as missing some sort of essential male characteristic. Having a friend ease them into it can go a long way toward making them more comfortable in the situation.

RESPONDING TO WHAT SUFFERERS SAY

"I have to exercise."

Don't attack the exercising. Just try to put it in context. For example, "I think it's great that you exercise, and I can see that you are getting wonderful results. But if you could take a break now and then, that could be a good thing for you as well."

"You're interfering with my schedule."

Maybe you can take "no" for an answer this time, but you don't have to take "no" for an answer every time. You might say, "You are so disciplined and consistent. I admire that. But I miss spending time with you. Don't you think it's okay to make time for other things in life? And for friends and family? To adjust our schedules sometimes? Life can get so rigid, but we don't have to let it."

Or, "Maybe now's not a good time, but I'm happy to shift my schedule around, too. Let's figure out when would be good."

"There's no way I can do this."

For the person who hasn't been exercising, getting started can be overwhelming. Reassure him that he can start small, with a short walk or some calisthenics. If he isn't up to that, he can learn how to do isometrics. He can do the kinds of exercises someone recovering from major surgery is given—simple movement initially done lying down. He can start with strength and stretching exercises and build a little endurance before adding any aerobic exercises such as walking. He can look into yoga and therapeutic classes conducted in pools.

The idea is to do a little more each day than the day before; it's not about doing something magnificent. You can say, "What can you do? Let's do that." Maybe it's walking to the mailbox; maybe it's walking to the end of the block; maybe it's building up to walking around the block; maybe it's parking farther and farther away.

Sometimes it helps to call it something else. Not exercise, but movement. Not exercise, but activity. It could be as simple as making minor changes in what she is already doing. She could think about all the things she does sitting down and try doing some of them standing up. Instead of waiting for things and people to come to her, she could go to them. That would entail more walking and carrying.

If he can afford it, or his insurance will pay, suggest that he work with a physical therapist or rehabilitation specialist for a few weeks. That will not only help get a routine established but will also help him quickly recognize some progress—which will help him maintain the routine and add to it once he's on his own.

The journey of a thousand miles begins with one step.

∞ —LAO TZU

Chapter Ten

Talking About Professional Help

∽

*I*t's easier to relax and not worry when you know that a professional is working with the person and the issues that concern you. This chapter covers:

- how to know someone is ready for help
- the types of professionals who might be of most assistance
- what professionals who work with eating disorders can do to help
- how to encourage someone to seek professional help
- what you can expect when someone goes for help
- how to talk about what is going on in treatment
- what to do when the help isn't helping
- what to do when someone refuses to go back

How do I know when to encourage professional help?

If you were concerned enough to purchase or read this book, you are probably dealing with a problem that could benefit from professional help. A professional can help you determine how significant the problem is, if the person you are worried about would benefit from treatment, or if it is something likely to resolve itself on its own.

Most eating disorders, like many other problems, are easier to deal with when they are just beginning. So seeing a professional early on has the potential to prevent small problems from turning into bigger ones.

Even if the problem has gone on for years, it's important to remember that hope helps. Talking about how a professional might be of assistance tells someone that "hope is on the way." This means that telling someone he needs professional help says that you believe that things can get better.

How can I tell if she is really ready to get help?

Most often she will tell you. She'll say things like, "You're right, I need help," or "I've got to do something different," or "I'm tired of suffering with this. I'm ready to deal with it." The classic line is, "I'm sick and tired of being sick and tired." Or some version on this same theme.

Often he will point out the things that most bother him. It might be, "I'm tired of being obsessed with food," "I don't want to go on another diet; I need something that will work for me this time," or "I wish I could find something that would help."

Take these statements as a sign that it is okay to talk about getting professional help. Say that you believe this would be a good idea and that you are happy about her decision to make things better.

Sometimes the desire for help fights with her fear that she is a failure because she has failed to solve this problem on her own. Stress that *she* isn't a failure and that considering help is often a first step in solving problems. Anything you can say about how you, or others you know, or have read about, got help and turned things around as a result is likely to be beneficial.

What will make him want to get help?

The main thing that drives a person to seek professional help is that he is suffering. Feeling bad is a powerful motivator. So it helps when you recognize and validate the suffering you see.

Keep in mind, though, that many people aren't ready to acknowledge that the reason for their suffering is their eating disorder. It is typical for them to locate the source of their pain in something else, such as feeling sick, being alone, not having friends, or having poor relationships with family or romantic partners. If the person you care about is in this type of denial, you don't have to confront the "real problem" to encourage help. You can encourage help for whatever problems he thinks he has.

Also, many people don't seek help because they are worried about how much it will cost and whether their insurance policy will pay. So help them look into what is covered; many insurance plans have some mental health or other provisions for dealing with eating disorders. Plus, not only can most professionals who work with eating disorders help you and the person you are concerned about determine the best alternatives, but also many hospitals, day treatment programs, and service providers have people on staff who can assist in determining the best way to pay for treatment.

Some people worry about the stigma associated with having a mental health problem. They may have heard people derided as "nutcases," "psychos," or "drama queens." If everyone who suffered was a "nutcase," we'd all be labeled. In reality all people suffer, and that doesn't make them "nutcases." It often helps to say something like, "The real 'nutcase' is the person who won't seek help," or "Most people respect people who have the courage to do something about the problems they have."

What types of professionals might help someone with an eating disorder?

Here is a list of some professionals and the qualifications they need to have in order to assess and treat the problems associated with having an eating disorder.

Medical Service Providers: are licensed by the state medical board to diagnose medical problems, physical problems, or mental health problems. They are also licensed to treat those problems with medication, physical manipulation, or medical advice. These physicians all take state boards that license them to practice medicine.

- MD's—Medical Doctors
- DO's—doctors of Osteopathic Medicine
- Psychiatrists are physicians, MD's or DO's, and are licensed to diagnose and treat mental illness including prescribing medication
- PA's—Physicians Assistants. Are licensed to provide medical services. Each state has different laws governing what they can

legally do. Here is a web page that provides information on a state by state basis for qualifications and scope of practice. http://www.aapa.org/gandp/statelaw.html

- NP's—Nurse Practitioner. Nurse with special training to practice under the supervision of a physician but who can prescribe medication and treatment. To find out more about what they are qualified to do you can look up this web page: http://www.womenshealthchannel.com/nursepractitioner.shtml.

Mental Health Professionals: Mental health professionals are licensed by the state to provide treatment for mental health problems. Not all mental health professionals are licensed to diagnose and treat without supervision. Each state has different licensing laws. Most often the following professionals are licensed to both diagnose and treat mental health problems:

- Psychiatrist (see above)
- Licensed Psychologists who have either a Ph.D., or Psy.D.(licensed to diagnose and treat mental illness—cannot prescribe medication) In most states this license is limited to professionals who have Doctorate degree in psychology, an internship, and two years of supervised experience. (And in a few states to those who have significant clinical experience and a Master's degree.)
- Licensed Professional Clinical Counselors (LPCC). (licensed to diagnose and treat mental illness—cannot prescribe medication). In most states this license is given to professionals with a minimum of a master's degree and three years of supervised experience.
- Licensed Clinical Social Workers (LCSW). (licensed to diagnose and treat mental illness—cannot prescribe medication). In most states this license is given to professionals with a minimum of a master's degree and three years of supervised experience.
- Licensed Marriage and Family Counselors (MFT) (MFCC). (licensed to treat marriage and family problems). In most states this license is supervised by the Board of Counseling and Social

Workers and is given to professionals who have a master's degree and several years of supervised experience.

If the person providing services is under supervision, they must disclose that information and those receiving services will have to sign a form saying they acknowledge that this information has been disclosed. The supervisor is responsible for all diagnoses and treatment plans.

Because the American Medical Association has assigned procedural codes for mental health services many insurance companies will pay for their services but only when they are provided by a licensed mental health professional. Some companies will only pay for mental health services provided by a psychologist or someone under their supervision. Others only pay for psychiatric services but that is rare.

Dieticians: Dieticians are also licensed, certified or registered by the state to provide nutrition services or advice to individuals requiring or seeking nutrition care or information. Only state-licensed, certified or registered dietetics professionals can provide nutrition counseling. States with certification laws limit the use of particular titles (eg, dietitian or nutritionist) to persons meeting predetermined requirements; however, persons not certified can still practice. You can find out about the requirements in your state by going to www.cdrnet.org/certifications/licensure/index.htm). The Commission on Dietetic Registration lists the following CDR certifications:

- Registered Dietitian: (RD)
- Dietetic Technician, Registered (DTR)
- Board Certified Specialist in Pediatric Nutrition (CSP)
- Board Certified Specialist in Renal Nutrition (CSR)
- Fellow of the American Dietetic Association (FADA)

Many insurance companies will pay for their services when they are provided by a licensed, registered, or certified specialist.

Since there are so many non-qualified sources of nutrition information and because most of us aren't familiar with the education and licensing requirements, it may help to check with your physician or licensed mental health professional about the necessary qualifications in your state for providing nutrition counseling for someone with an eating disorder.

Athletic Trainers: Forty-three states license athletic trainers. These highly skilled health care professionals must pass an examination and hold a bachelors degree to become an:

- ATC. Athletic Trainer, Certified. Over 70 percent of athletic trainers also have a masters degree. Athletic trainers practice under the direction of physicians and can assist in risk management and injury prevention, therapeutic exercise, assessment and evaluation, acute care of injury and illness, and treatment and rehabilitation for physically active people.

Exercise Physiologists: The American Society of Exercise Physiologists accredits academic programs to graduate professionals with degrees in Exercise Physiology. After completing an academic program these professionals can take an ASEP exam to become certified EPCs:

- Certified Exercise Physiologist, Bachelors degree EPCs often work as program coordinators for fitness programs.
- Masters degree EPCs often direct exercise programs within clinical and fitness settings.
- PhD degree EPCs often coordinate research and teaching in universities and colleges. Depending on their training and background they can be a good source of information on exercise for well people. If they have additional training and experience with eating disorders they might be helpful in designing a workable exercise regimen.

Dentists: Dentists are also licensed by the state. Many people with eating disorders have dental problems. First, vomiting produces damage to the enamel on the teeth. Second, the gums, teeth, and mouth have distinctive features when someone is malnourished.

Do the credentials of a health care professional matter?

Yes. State license boards are set up to protect the public. They govern what health care professionals can do, and they oversee the process of making sure each professional has the training to provide the services the credentialing board oversees. Years of research have gone into determining what kinds of experience and education a professional needs in order to practice effectively and safely. In addition, the license board investigates and can take action against a professional who has harmed a client. When people advertise themselves as professionals but are not governed by license boards, they cannot be held responsible for what they call themselves or what services they provide.

What form does treatment for eating disorders take?

There are a variety of ways treatment is delivered. Many combine exercise, art therapy, music therapy, nutrition counseling, and vocational counseling. These range from full-time hospital care, to day treatment programs, to outpatient individual or group sessions. Some treatment facilities employ a full range of professionals on site. Other professionals work in consultation with each other even if they aren't in the same facility.

Some programs emphasize individual sessions. Some use both individual and group therapies. Group therapy, both outpatient and in a hospital setting, is popular and can be effective. On the other hand, it has certain limitations. Comparing themselves to other group members can intensify some people's problems. For example, people suffering from anorexia are often overwhelmed by seeing others who are thinner. People with bulimia can learn new techniques from others in the group and get worse. But many people with compulsive overeating have benefited from finding out that they are not alone and have learned helpful ways to avoid the pitfalls of troublesome behavior patterns.

It is important for you not to make recommendations about which approach might be best. The professionals dealing with the situation need to make those judgments. And even when your feelings about the type of treatment being provided conflicts with what the person you care about is getting, it's best to keep quiet on these matters if you can.

If you are worried you can ask the person receiving treatment, "Are you okay with how your treatment is working?" or "How do you feel about the way this is going for you?"

What might make it necessary to intervene?

There are several situations that make it necessary to intervene. If treatment is being delivered by someone without adequate credentials you should questioned it. If the person you are concerned about has a sexual relationship with the treatment provider, if there is touching that makes the person you are worried about upset, or if the treatment seems bizarre, you need to say something. "I know you feel desperate, but do you really think this treatment plan makes sense? It seems strange to me." Saying something this strong is fine so long as you are willing to back off if you are met with disagreement. If you are really concerned about what you are hearing, call the licensing board for that professional and ask if this is a reasonable way to treat the problems at hand. If the professional seems to be practicing without a license, that too can be reported. For example, if someone is providing medical advice without a medical degree, contact the state board for physicians.

How do you know which type of professional to look for?

Encourage the person you are concerned about to select a professional who can target the problems she is most concerned about. For example, if she says, "I don't even know how to eat anymore; I'm so mixed-up with all these diets," a dietician is most likely to have the information that will engage her in getting better. But if she says, "I can't stand feeling obsessed with food all the time; I can't think about anything else," perhaps a mental health professional might be most helpful. On the other hand, if she is concerned because she keeps vomiting even when she doesn't want to, perhaps a physician would be the first person to contact.

If the professional you contact is experienced with eating disorders, he or she will be able to put you and the person you are worried about in contact with other professionals who could help with associated problems. Many people who regularly work with eating disorders take a multidisciplinary team approach. Therefore, they'll know professionals from other disciplines and they'll know how they can move these problems forward toward workable solutions.

Should I set up the first appointment?

It's not a good idea to set up an actual appointment yourself, because the effort involved in setting up the appointment is a good indicator that the person who has the problem is ready to follow through. You can express your concern and then offer your assistance in locating a professional who has experience with eating disorders. (However, if you are the parent of a minor child, you will not only need to set up the appointment; you will also have to provide permission for that treatment.)

What are some of the medical problems associated with eating disorders?

Because these problems are so interrelated, we'll list the major medical complications for eating disorders in one section. (19.)

- Malnutrition: A deficiency in micronutrients that can be caused by undereating, overeating, or avoiding certain food groups such as carbohydrates, fats, vegetables, or protein. This can lead to problems such as excessive fatigue, infections, kidney problems, and heart abnormalities.
- Dehydration: Lack of adequate hydration can lead to electrolyte imbalances. Electrolytes are essential to the body's "natural electricity" that ensures healthy teeth, joints, and bones, nerve and muscle impulses, kidneys and heart, blood-sugar levels, and delivery of oxygen to the cells.
- Hyponatremia: This dangerous condition can lead to fluid in the lungs, brain swelling, nausea, vomiting, and confusion. It is caused by drinking too much water or "water loading" (typically more than eight eight-ounce glasses in a twelve-hour period).
- Edema: Swelling of the soft tissue as a result of excess water accumulation (can be caused by laxative and diuretic abuse).
- Muscle atrophy: Wasting away of muscle, which can include the heart.

- Impaired neuromuscular function: This is a result of vitamin and mineral deficiencies, usually potassium.
- Insomnia: Hunger can keep people awake.
- Hypotension: Low blood pressure causes low body temperature, malnutrition, and dehydration. Can lead to heart arrhythmias, shock, or myocardial infarction.
- Orthostatic hypotension: A sudden drop in blood pressure when standing up which can lead to dizziness, blurred vision, passing out, heart pounding, and headaches.
- Disruptions in blood sugar: Can lead to problems with liver, kidneys, and neurological functioning.
- Osteoporosis: Thinning of the bones. The body seeks sources of calcium from the bones when the diet is deficient in calcium.
- Vitamin deficiencies: Decreases the body's ability to heal itself, which can cause skin that bruises easily, low blood pressure, low platelet count.
- Bad circulation, slowed or irregular heartbeat, arrhythmias, angina, heart attack: Electrolyte imbalances (especially from potassium deficiency, dehydration, or malnutrition) place extra strain on the heart muscle.
- Hyperactivity: Not being able to slow down and relax; constant motion or activity.
- Swelling in the face and neck: Glands can swell as a result of self-induced vomiting.
- Gastrointestinal bleeding: Bleeding in the digestive tract.
- Mallory-Weiss tear: A tear of the gastro-esophageal junction associated with vomiting.
- Digestive difficulties: Ulcers, deficiencies in digestive enzymes that lead the body to have difficulty digesting and absorbing nutrients.
- Ketoacidosis: High levels of acids build up in the blood (known as ketosis), caused by the body burning fat (instead of sugar and carbohydrates) to get energy. Many dieters restrict carbohydrates in order to achieve this condition, but there are health consequences of maintaining this practice.
- Depression and anxiety

- Tooth decay and gum disease
- Tear of the esophagus
- Acid reflux
- Irritable bowel
- Headaches and fatigue

Do these symptoms mean that emergency action is required?

If the condition is severe and causing significant distress, a medical evaluation is necessary to determine whether an immediate intervention is necessary. Chapter twelve covers what to do, when to do it, and how to go about it.

What can I say when I observe these symptoms?

Don't panic when you read this list of possible medical complications for eating disorders. It does not mean that everyone with an eating disorder will develop all these problems. In fact, most people who have eating disorders get better before these conditions develop. Nonetheless, many people do develop physical problems that need to be addressed.

This list makes clear that there is a strong "mind–body" connection between health problems and eating problems. For example, someone might start restricting what she eats because her boyfriend left her for someone else. She feels lonely, sad, and depressed. However, the lack of food will also produce additional symptoms, such as not being able to sleep, feeling light-headed, and certainly feeling fatigued. After a while it's hard to tell what is causing what.

What you can do is express your concern. Mention what you have observed, assure him that you care, and say you can see the suffering these problems seem to be causing. Then encourage him to try professional help with someone who has experience with eating disorders.

Don't some people with eating disorders need to be in a hospital?

Some do. But *you* don't have to make that decision. The decision to put someone in a hospital to treat an eating disorder should be made by a physician or a mental health professional, together with the person who has the problem. However, if the person you are concerned about has a significant health problem or is talking about suicide, you should take them to an emergency room to be evaluated. (This is covered in more detail in chapter twelve.)

How can a medical doctor help?

Most people who have eating disorders would like to believe that what they are doing will not have long-term consequences. They don't realize that prolonged self-induced vomiting will create mouth, throat and digestive-tract problems, or that compulsive overeating will lead them to the medical risks associated with obesity. A consultation with a doctor can bring some of this home to them.

Encouraging medical help can be like offering water to a thirsty person stranded in the desert. When someone is struggling with an eating disorder they can believe there is no way out. They are often embarrassed because they see themselves as someone who knows better but is somehow caught in an awful trap. A physician can make clear the health risks associated with most eating disorders and at the same time reassure them that there is a way out.

If you are a parent, guardian, or someone else, like a coach, who has the prerogative to require a medical exam, that is probably a good idea. But keep in mind that a quick physical when the physician has not been alerted to the eating disorder may end up being a waste of money. Make sure that the physician you select knows which medical tests might provide information about the consequences of having disordered eating.

How can a mental health professional help?

Most people who have eating disorders also have problems with depression, anxiety, substance abuse, post-traumatic stress disorder, or other adjustment problems. It's often hard to know which came first. But whether the eating disorder creates other mental health concerns or the mental health problems produce the eating disorder, the fact remains that both need to be treated. Otherwise the person you care about may simply trade one set of symptoms for another.

Mental knots are a significant part of all eating disorders. People with these problems want to please, but feel conflicted about taking care of basic personal needs while also meeting the assumed demands of society, family, friends, and lovers. A mental health professional can often help the person who is suffering see how dieting, overexercising, eating too much or not enough, vomiting, or whatever else won't really mend what is wrong. In addition, he can offer compassionate understanding of the pain and the desperation that develop as a result of having a problem others judge harshly, and then can assess how to move forward with solutions.

Some problems are so hard to deal with that people get so overwhelmed that they bury their turmoil in thinking about food and weight. Think about trying to fix a car that isn't working. The person with an eating disorder is focused on fixing a flat tire when the real problem is in the carburetor. When the eating disorder seems like the only way to deal with life, a therapist can help figure out why these symptoms began, what sustains these problems, and how to find ways other than the eating disorder to take care of what is wrong. In this way, a trained mental health professional can help the person who is suffering discover why the eating disorder seems like a solution instead of a problem.

For example, Ned developed his eating disorder when he was seventeen and his parents were going through a divorce. He had a lot of anger and sadness that he found hard to express, and neither parent was available to hear the pain he felt. Instead, he worked out extensively; he dieted and built muscle. This intense activity allowed him to not focus on his *real* pain. When his dieting and overexercising led him to the point of exhaustion and he could no longer exercise so much, he had to face his feelings of depression and sadness. He had focused his problem on his body, assuming that his lack of muscle tone was making him lack confidence. Therapy helped him to see that his problem was not his body (the tire); it was his sadness, loss, and anger over the divorce (the carburetor). Once he started working on the right problem, he was able to get better.

How can a dietician help?

Many people with eating disorders don't know how to eat in a nutritious way. Others know what to do but can't get themselves to do it. They have tried one diet plan after another and have often only ended up with more problems. A dietician who is skilled with eating disorders not only knows what changes need to be made to adequately fuel a body, but even more important, she can help pace the changes so as not to overwhelm the person who is already terrified of changing eating habits.

Many people with eating disorders will say things like, "I have no idea what normal eating is. I think I'm eating too much (or too little), but I can't tell anymore." A dietician skilled in working with eating disorders can help pace the introduction of new foods as well as the withdrawal of some old favorites.

What can an exercise physiologist or athletic trainer do to help someone with an eating disorder?

Whether someone is exercising too much because they're scared of gaining weight or worried they can't exercise because they are too overweight, an exercise consultant can help figure out an efficient plan. Many overexercisers aren't getting the benefits that exercise can provide. Instead they are wearing themselves out and overtaxing their muscles, which can only lead to injury and discomfort. Many overexercisers are surprised to discover that less is actually more when weight training is balanced with aerobic activity and the body has periods of rest that allow muscle to develop.

Likewise many underexercisers are scared off because they believe they can't exercise enough to make a difference. They are often delighted to know that walking ten minutes can matter.

Maybe you have said as much before and felt frustrated because your advice wasn't heard. It helps to remember the last time you were also slow to pay attention to useful advice and had to be told something a number of times before it finally clicked. It is often an offhand comment or a tip from a professional that tips the "can-do" scale. A professional has experience not only with what exercise routine is likely to work for each individual; he also has experience motivating people to try things they never thought possible.

What's a good way to bring up the idea of seeing a professional?

There are better and worse ways to open this conversation. And depending on how grave the situation seems to you, you might want to float some feelers and then back off for a while. Bring up the subject again a few days later and, depending on your relationship, persevere and push a little harder after a little more time has elapsed.

To open the conversation, it helps to point out what you have observed. You might try something such as:

- "You seem to have lost some color in your face. Are you feeling okay?"
- "Your skin's a little flushed today. Are you okay?"
- "I remember when you seemed happier."
- "I worry about you; you seem on edge."

Any suggestion for professional help will go better if the person you are worried about has acknowledged that he is suffering, that he'd like to find better ways to cope, and that he is tired of struggling with these problems without getting much better. Sometimes it's useful to say that you are aware that he has suffered enough by saying:

- "It's hard to watch you suffer with this."
- "No matter what, I'm here for you, but I wish you would think about talking to a professional too."
- "You've struggled with this long enough. Do you think it's time to try something else?"
- "Professionals talk to lots of people who share these same problems. I'm guessing they might have some new things you could try."
- "There are always different ways to look at these problems. Perhaps a professional could shed some new light on this."

But you'll also need to be prepared to back off when the person you wish would get help doesn't make that appointment. Down the road you can bring it up again when she seems more receptive or when she is again talking about how her problems are difficult to deal with on her own.

When you bring up the topic again at another time, you could be a little more direct:

- "I know you seem to like that thin look; to me it doesn't seem healthy."
- "I'm worried that you're not getting around as well. And you seem short on energy."
- "I've noticed that you don't seem to be able to concentrate as well. That was always your strong suit. What do you think might be going on?"
- "You don't seem to have time for the things you used to do. Is it that you don't enjoy them anymore or is it something else?"

The next time, you might connect the dots:

- "I think you've more than pushed the envelope here."
- "I wish you didn't feel you had to be perfect. Do you think you could stand me if I were perfect?"
- "Can we talk about why you don't believe me when I tell you I think you look(ed) great?"
- "I think this has gone beyond lifestyle choices. I think your weight (gain/loss) is affecting your health."
- "You seem to be eating a lot more, yet you don't seem to be getting a lot of satisfaction from it. Are you under a lot of stress? Is there anything I can do?"
- "We never grab a meal together anymore. I miss it. What did I do?"
- "Hey, I know you've been having a lot of problems with school-work, family, other stuff. Maybe you'd feel comfortable talking to someone about it. I might know someone. . . . I think you'll feel better."

And then you can be direct and suggest that the person you care about seek some answers, some guidance, some actual help:

- "I just can't dance around this any longer. I'm really worried about you."
- "Maybe it's happened so gradually that you can't see it, and since I don't see you every day I can. You've lost (gained) so

much weight. Something is wrong. What are you doing to get a handle on it?"

- "I can see that something has really changed in your life. Your routines are different. You look different. Yet you don't seem happy. And you don't seem to feel well. Have you thought about seeing a doctor and getting a checkup?"

And most important, you might need to say, "Something is wrong here and I think you need help."

In addition, you might put a name to what you see and offer to find help.

- "You've lost a lot of weight. I'm concerned you might have lost too much. That might make you vulnerable to every bug that comes around. But more than that, I'm worried that you may be sliding into an eating disorder. It's really hard to get out of this problem once you're in it. I wish you'd talk to someone about whether you're in danger of doing that, how to tell, and how to avoid it."
- "I'm scared that you might be on the verge of developing an eating disorder. I've known people who've been there, and it's very tough on the mind as well as the body. The more it gets entrenched, the harder and longer it takes to recover. Do you know someone you could consult to figure out if that's what's happening? If you are uncomfortable, maybe there are places for confidential screenings. I could look into it if you want."
- "I can see that the way you are eating has led to the weight you've been putting on, and that seems to be getting in your way. I care and I'm scared that it will affect your health. It is putting such a strain on your heart. I don't think it is just regular eating and indulging anymore. I think it might be more than that. Please find someone who knows about these things and check it out. If this is an eating disorder, the sooner you do something about it, the better off you'll be. I want you healthy and happy in the long term, not just for right now."
- "I'm scared that something is happening to you, and I'm scared that it might be an eating disorder. Maybe that sounds crazy,

but that's what I think. I wish you would check it out. It's not the kind of thing people can recover from on their own."

- "Eating disorders are dangerous and hurtful. I don't want you to be injured or harmed."
- "I've had an eating disorder myself and am still dealing with the consequences. You know that (or I don't know if you knew that). I don't know exactly what you are going through, but I suggest you see someone so you don't have any further health problems down the line. Please think about it."

How can I find a professional?

There are a variety of ways to find a professional.

- recommendations from trusted friends
- referral from a physician
- crisis hotlines
- child protective services
- school, college, and university counseling centers
- community mental health agencies
- clergy
- employee assistance programs
- emergency services (fire, police, rescue)
- hospitals
- state psychological associations, or state counselor associations
- associations for registered dieticians (American Dietetic Association)
- other professional associations for athletic trainers, exercise physiologists, medical professions
- National Eating Disorders Association

The person you care about may not know the best way to find out if a certain professional has experience with eating disorders. So encourage him to ask directly. You should also encourage him to find out if this professional *likes* to work with these problems; some professionals have experience but prefer not to work with eating disorders.

What if he already has a professional he likes but she doesn't have experience with eating disorders?

Some professionals are comfortable working with eating disorders and others are not. Doctors who expect immediate change or who believe that telling a patient what to do is sufficient to solve an eating problem are often frustrated when working with these problems. That frustration is usually picked up by the person suffering, and that can lead him to pretend that everything is okay when it isn't.

Encourage the person you're worried about to ask his doctor for a referral to someone who does have experience with eating disorders.

What if I bring up getting help and she says she can handle this on her own?

Many, if not most, people who suffer from eating disorders wish they could just decide to change and then fix their problems by themselves. Feeling this way is understandable. So you'll want to acknowledge that this desire to take care of themselves by themselves is a good thing. But you'll also want to find some ways to encourage getting help.

You can acknowledge their motivation to get better with comments such as:

- "I'm really glad that you want to feel better."
- "I'm glad you have some ideas about what you can do."
- "It takes a lot of courage to think about changing."
- "I admire what you are trying to do."

Acknowledging that she wants to take care of herself in her own way doesn't mean that you can't bring up professional help later, when she seems more receptive to that idea.

But pushing someone to get help when she doesn't want to won't work, even when she needs it desperately. Most of us who are hoping for change count on just getting the person we're worried about in the door of a professional, who will then take over and convince her that she needs help. Sometimes this works, but more frequently the person who is suffering will go to the professional and deny the problem, or defend the problem by saying things like, "It's only temporary," or "It's not really bothering me that much." Then she'll come back to you and tell you that the professional "said I don't have a problem."

Sometimes people come for help because they have been given an ultimatum: "You either go for help or else . . ." Again, this usually won't work. If the person who is suffering isn't ready to talk to a professional, he will go just long enough to convince you that he is sincere about wanting you not to worry. That consideration is not what you are hoping for. You want him to pursue treatment because he knows he needs it. But in this case he is likely to go for you, not for the problems that are causing so much discomfort.

On the bright side, sometimes the push to consult a professional leads the person suffering with an eating disorder to conclude that "people are worried enough to think I need professional help—so maybe I really do." Other times the person with the eating disorder has been considering professional help, and your suggestion is just the boost they need to actually make the appointment. When the concern of others resonates with their own concerns it can reinforce their desire to get better and suffer less. As professionals will tell you, it is often the push by a friend or relative that is the primary motivation for making the initial appointment.

What role should I take in trying to find professional help?

You don't want to push, force, or coerce someone into doing things he is not ready to do. On the other hand, that doesn't mean you should sit back and do nothing when someone says he wants professional help. Be guided by the person you care about; ask how you can best help with this process.

Does she want you to find resources such as books? That's a great way to help, and we have listed some at the end of this book. Identifying a local professional who has experience working with eating disorders is also something you can help out with. On the other hand, encouraging them to look for their own resources will strengthen their commitment to actually following through with getting help.

What if you have located resources and the person you wish would get help says things like, "Oh, no, I can't go *there* . . ." or "Yes, but I've heard that doesn't work," or "Can't you find something that wouldn't mean I'd have to . . . ?" Recognize that he is worried about making changes and is likely to find strong reasons to resist pursuing *any* sources of help that seem threatening. Rationalizations that begin with "yes, but" usually mean he isn't ready to pursue it, so don't try to answer his objections. Ask first if he wants your help, encourage when it seems appropriate, and then back off when his ambivalence about getting help swings toward "not right now."

Should I go to his first appointment?

Some people feel cared about and supported when you go with them and are right there afterward. These gestures can strengthen relationships and enhance bonds.

Others feel like they want to "go it alone" to show that they can manage.

The key here is not to make yourself a part of the equation. You don't want to feel like you are not important if you are not included, or that your going or not going is evidence of the overall importance of your relationship. Keep the focus on what is most beneficial to the person who is trying to figure out how to get the help he needs.

Should I ask about how it went?

Once someone goes for help, it's natural to be curious about how it all went. You'll want to know if she liked her therapist, or if she learned anything new, or if she plans to do something different.

The fact is, most people walk out of any therapy session, whether with a dietician, physician, or a mental health professional, with a lot to absorb, and most often they're not sure what they should do next. Having to talk about what they think right after an appointment is hard, because they need time to digest what happened. First they have to think about what they think; then they need to figure out what they want you to know; and, most important, they usually don't want to upset you with what they are learning.

So don't probe. Instead, you might say:

- "I'm glad you went. If you want to talk, I'm willing."
- "I can imagine that it is hard to digest all that's happened; perhaps now isn't a good time to talk about it."

- "If you want to talk, I'm ready. If not, that's okay too."
- "I care about what you are learning and how you feel. Let me know when and if you'd like to talk."
- "I can imagine you have a lot to sort through. If and when you want to talk, I'm open. Meanwhile, what would you like to do (or talk about)?"
- "I care about what is happening to you, and I'm open to hearing about it when you are ready."

What if she wants to talk and I'm not ready?

If you are too emotional or upset about this or anything else, just be up front that you're not up to listening.

- "Now isn't a good time for me. Perhaps we could talk later."
- "I can't focus on this now, but I want you to know that I'll be more open when . . ."
- "I can't really talk about this now, but I could talk about other things."
- "Just because I can't talk now doesn't mean I don't care. I do."

What if she won't talk about seeing a professional?

Some people won't acknowledge they have a problem. Others will feel that what they are doing is sufficient to solve the problem. Most will feel you are being intrusive if you push. So if you can, back off and wait for another time to bring this topic up.

What if he tells me, "You're all I need. I don't want to talk to anyone else"?

This is clearly the time to bring up your limitations in terms of knowledge, time, and patience. Promising to listen and be there to help without expressing those limitations can end up being a trap for both of you. Though you might feel flattered that you have been selected as a confidant and helper, keep in mind how frustrated you are apt to become when things don't improve in the way you would like.

Point out that "you would never consider letting me fix your broken arm," "decide what the prescription should be for your glasses," or "represent you in court." Professionals know that eating disorders take a long time to turn around, and they are prepared to handle the inevitable setbacks. Because professionals don't have a personal stake in the outcome, they can remain more objective. And most important, a professional has the benefit of years of experience working with eating disorders. You can point out all these reasons why a professional is a better alternative than relying on friends or family for recovering from an eating disorder.

Along these lines, it might help to say:

- "I wish I could be there to help with this, but frankly it's over my head. I feel frustrated because I know I don't have the skills to help you with this problem."
- "I appreciate your confidence in me. It means a lot. But you need to appreciate that I don't have the skills to help you with this problem. I'd feel better if you also saw a professional who could really help. I'll still be here."
- "Even if you see a professional, you need to know that I'll be here for you, caring and listening. I just want you to realize that I feel bad when I know someone with professional experience would really be of more benefit to you."
- "You always say you should find the best person possible for the job at hand. Unfortunately, I'm not that person."

If the person you are worried about resists these suggestions, repeat that you have limits in terms of time, patience, and resources. And be prepared to have this conversation more than once. Each time he says, "You're the only one who cares," reiterate that you can't take on this responsibility and that professionals are in a better position to know what needs to be done to help.

What if I don't think the clinic/therapists know what they are doing?

Be extremely careful about expressing doubt about someone's therapy. It can make him feel confused, insecure, unsafe, and can distract him from the focus he needs as he dedicates himself to getting better.

Suggesting that you don't have faith in the treatment he is receiving can undermine progress. You also have to realize that you may not be in a position to judge accurately. You might be misinterpreting behavior. You might have unrealistic expectations. You might assume the process should be going faster or more smoothly. It might seem as if the person you care about is pulling away from you, and you might be reacting to that without realizing it.

Perhaps the best you can do in this circumstance is ask the person you are worried about what *she* thinks of the help she is getting. If she doesn't think she's making progress, ask why. Is it the therapist? Is it her motivation? Is something else getting in the way?

What should I say if she doesn't like her therapist?

If the relationship just doesn't click, encourage her to consult a different therapist. There are many skilled practitioners who have experience with eating disorders, and while one may not suit, another might seem just right. But it can also be helpful to talk about what the problem might be. Maybe what the therapist says seems too intrusive or is hard to understand. Point out that therapists, no matter how skilled, can't read minds, and that if the process isn't going well, most good therapists will be receptive to talking about what is not working.

Is it ever a good idea to take a break from therapy if it seems too hard?

Yes. People need to work when they are ready. Sometimes people resist therapy because the therapist is pushing too hard, too soon. It helps to know they can step back if they need to. Most people who want to make changes do so over a period of time that includes breaks. Sometimes a person suffering from an eating disorder needs to concentrate on something else, like taking an exam, caring for a sick child, or finishing a project. Let the person you are concerned about know that you won't stop caring because she stops therapy. Some people with eating disorders fear that if they aren't thinking about this problem every second they won't get better. But that's the way they burn out on their treatment. If you notice this happening, suggest talking to her therapist about the possibility of taking a break.

Part III

∞

SPECIAL ISSUES: GOING THE DISTANCE

*M*ost childhood problems don't result from "bad" parenting.

∞—FRED ROGERS

Chapter Eleven

Talking to Young People

∽

*T*rying to understand their own or someone else's eating disorder is challenging enough for adults with years of experience; it's even more difficult for young people. Young people are vulnerable. And it is their great asset—their openness—which makes them vulnerable to the pressures of friends and the media. But that openness also makes it possible for us to help them sort things out and juggle the inevitable cultural pressures.

Young people, like the rest of us, need support to tackle these tough problems. They may not have the experience to manage their feelings. As the adults in their lives, we need to provide more guidance and take more action when we see them harming themselves. Keep in mind, that strict age markers don't mean as much as general maturity and responsibility. If the person you are worried about is eighteen, but still somewhat immature and not able to take clear responsibility for good self-care, this chapter can help you figure out what to say and do.

It will help you answer two fundamental questions: how to talk to children who have a parent, sibling, or other loved one who is suffering from an eating disorder, and how to talk to a child or teen who may be developing an eating disorder. Some of it will apply to young children, some to teens, and some to both. Keep in mind that much of what is suggested in the rest of this book can be adapted to children, too.

What should we say when someone they know has an eating disorder?

Helping a child understand what *we're* having trouble understanding is a challenge that is best met with honesty. Children cope best when they are told what is happening and what they can do to help. We don't want to say too much and overwhelm a small child, but we also know that not saying enough can leave them grasping for answers. And because children often come up with unreasonable, fanciful, and frightening ideas about what they don't comprehend, we need to help them understand and cope. When you are not sure what to say, it helps to try out your ideas on someone else first, someone who can give you feedback about adjusting your words to the maturity level of the child.

Tell the child that the person:

- is having trouble
- will eventually get better, and that you are all hopeful things will improve over time
- is like many other people whose families struggle to figure out ways to cope and still have good lives
- is coping with life's problems in a way that is not working so well, and that these problems are causing her to suffer
- is not a good role model to follow when it comes to eating
- needs some special attention and time, but that just because you (the child) are not currently suffering does not mean your needs are unimportant
- is not more important than you are

It also helps to reassure a child that he:

- has no responsibility for the development of this problem
- can be considerate and compassionate by not expecting quick changes
- can continue to have a good relationship with the person he is concerned about, even though that person is having a hard time

- doesn't need to discuss the problems she is worried about if she doesn't want to
- can ask you about the problems he is observing
- is not necessarily going to develop the same problems

Most important, you want to make sure you have left the door open for questions later on by saying things such as, "If you think of things later that you want to talk about, be sure and let me know," or "I want you to know that you can ask questions about this anytime you have them."

The worst thing to do is to leave the young person in the dark. Children younger than three care about others, sense when something isn't right, and also pick up tension in the family. We need to care about what they are sensing, learning, and feeling.

A lot of young children know more than they let on. They may act as though they have no idea that someone else in the family is suffering, either because they don't want to further upset the family or because they assume they should go along with the denial that they see around them. But that doesn't mean that they haven't noticed that others are suffering and that the ways that they are suffering are leading them to act in weird ways. If you talk to them about it, you reassure them and, equally important, help them acquire important life lessons.

What can you say about someone with an eating disorder?

You can say things such as:

- "Your mom has a problem with eating; have you noticed?"
- "What have you noticed about ___?"
- "What do you think about what she is doing?"

Reinforce the realistic and compassionate things that children so often say. When they are judgmental or harsh, help them soften their view by pointing out kinder ways to interpret what they are observing. Also help them understand that they shouldn't take things that are happening personally. For example:

- "Your mom is not avoiding the dinner table because she doesn't like us. She is struggling to figure some things out, and we need to be nice to her while she is working on this problem."
- "Right now your sister is totally focused on her weight, which isn't really a problem, so she continues to worry about the wrong thing. We need to be patient with her while she tries to figure this out."
- "Your mother and I are doing what we can to help your brother, and we are confident this will get better. Right now you need to know that you don't have to worry about this."
- "I know it is hard to hear, 'Do as I say, not as I do.' I realize what I'm doing isn't a good idea, and I'm working on changing, but meanwhile my hope is that you will continue to do the good, healthy things you are currently doing. That's what you need to do. And that's great."
- "The nicest thing we can do for each other in this family is to take good care of ourselves, even when we notice others are having a hard time."

Should I say something about a bad habit my child is noticing?

Yes. Trying to rationalize strange behavior only confuses young children. It's better to just fess up and say, "Yeah, that's not a good idea"; "You're right, what your sister is doing isn't healthy"; "I'm glad you can see that what your mom is doing probably isn't a good way to exercise," and you can add, "but we need to be patient while she tries to figure this out."

If someone in the family has an eating disorder, do the other children need to go to the therapy?

Some young people are profoundly reluctant to talk to strangers (therapists) about personal matters. But if they are worried about what is happening to their parent or sibling, talking to a professional can help them better understand what their loved one is going through and be reassured that things will be okay in time.

If the whole family is in therapy, should I force a child who is reluctant to go to participate?

That would be something to talk to the therapist about; perhaps there are reasons why she wants the whole family to be there, or maybe it isn't necessary. Usually the therapist will give you some advice on how to involve reluctant family members.

What should I do if I think my child may be developing an eating disorder?

If you are worried about the ways that your child is eating or not eating and think he might be developing an eating disorder, talk with your family physician, pediatrician, or a mental health professional who is knowledgeable about normal child development.

You should not try to figure this out by yourself. It is frustrating. It's scary. And you don't have to face these difficult dilemmas alone. There are many professionals skilled in helping you figure out whether or not your child has a problem, and what you can say or do to improve the chances of solving these problems.

Should I talk to him about what I notice?

Yes, it's important to point out what you are noticing. It's also a good idea to say you are worried and that you will have to seek help to make sure that your child is safe and not in medical danger. You can say:

- "Good parents have to do something when they notice problems, and we're (or I'm) concerned about what you are doing."
- "You may think you are okay, but it's not okay to ___."
- "I know you think this is a good idea, I want you to know that even if we disagree, it's important to me that we keep talking about this. So, I'll tell you what I think, and you tell me what you think."
- "It's hard to watch you suffer with this; I think we should get some help, what do you think?"
- "Your suffering like this is not okay with me. I have to do something to make sure you are healthy."

- "Just because I think this is a problem doesn't mean I'm disappointed in you. All young people have problems and it's a parent's job to help them out. Please don't close me out."

Should I talk to her about it a lot?

No. In your day-to-day interactions, it is better to back off and help her find more areas in which she can have control. This is especially important for teens, because they are not yet living independently. So much of their day is programmed by someone else, and so much of where they need to be, what they need to do, and when they need to do it are dictated by other people, too. Also, when she can focus on things other than eating, she can redirect her energy. Getting a pet, taking up a new hobby, joining a new club, getting involved in a cause: anything that is time-consuming, social, and rewarding.

Where are all the moods and demands coming from?

When someone is preoccupied with food and then how to get rid of it, there is little room for anything else. And since they know that most other people would be upset with their thinking, they get defensive and then angry. Even before you have tried to talk them out of what they are doing, their frustration and tension can become too big to hold in. Because they trust that you care for them, they may feel safe to go beyond venting—to hurting you in what they say and do. And because they can't see how to give up the eating disorder, they may make incredible demands, and because they sometimes believe that their failure to get better is your fault for not being accommodating enough, they lash out. But as we discussed in chapter three on setting limits, meeting their unreasonable demands won't help.

What are some things I should avoid saying?

Young people sense criticism even when we don't intend to be critical or judgmental. When we are frustrated it is easy to justify our responses by saying, "I was only being honest." It helps to keep in mind that a lot of damage can be done in the name of "honesty". Sometimes the better choice is to hold back on what you honestly think. This is even more true with young people than with adults, because they are so vulnerable to what other people think of them. Here are some things to be particularly careful of. These are things that still resonate years later in an adult's mind, even if they were only kids when they felt the anger, confusion, and pain from hearing someone say:

- "I can't believe you are doing this to yourself."
- "Don't you realize you are killing yourself?"
- "If you don't stop this you'll put your mother in a mental hospital."
- "If you loved me, you would . . ."
- "After all we've done for you, how can you . . ."
- "If you don't stop eating those stupid snacks, you'll end up fat."
- "If you eat like that, you'll have a heart attack before you are thirty."
- "You need to set a better example for your younger sister."
- "You'll never have children if you don't stop this."
- "Until you get some help with this, you're grounded."
- "Your getting better is going to make this family so much better."
- "I can't believe you could think this was a good idea."
- "Stop hiding from your problems; you've got to face this thing squarely."
- "You can lick this; stop your whining and get on with it."

Once you stop to think about these comments it's easy to see how they could be taken the wrong way. But there are a number of other things we say to be helpful, to show support, or just to make conversation that can backfire. Here are some of those and the reasons why they don't work.

"Oh, look, you finished everything on your plate. You must have been really hungry."
These comments can make a person with anorexia feel about three years old. They don't want people commenting on their eating habits any more than you or I do.

"Are you sure you want to leave that on your plate?"
It is not helpful to ask someone who has anorexia this question, because chances are she does want to leave it there. And your question

may make her feel she has to work harder to hide the fact that she isn't eating. So she may eat and spit the food out in a napkin, or get more creative about getting it to the dog or somewhere else.

If he has bulimia, this only reinforces the notion that people are watching what he eats. If he is struggling with obesity, it only draws attention to his decision to forgo what's there and can magnify the temptation to eat it anyway.

"Your mother went to a lot of trouble fixing this meal; you'd better eat it."

You're hoping a little guilt will help, and it may seem to work well. But guilt fuels eating disorders and can make the sufferer more likely to retreat, isolate herself, and then cut herself off from what she most needs—our compassion and understanding. Rather then going for guilt, try saying what you expect. For example, "In this house we expect you to be at the dinner table. You don't have to eat, but you need to show up, because this is how our family stays connected."

"You'll end up like ___ if you keep eating like that."

Usually when we say this, it's because we are worried that he could develop the same problems as another family member. But he won't hear worry. What he hears is that you expect to be disappointed in him in the future, or that you already are disappointed. A young child will think you are angry and hear that "I'm on the way to disappointing the family, just like ___." We don't want that to happen.

"Are you sure you want to eat ___?"

You're trying to be helpful, but this question isn't really a question; it's a criticism. What she hears is that she shouldn't eat what she has in front of her. Unless you have been told, "Tell me when you think I'm just eating for some reason other than hunger," it's best to keep your observation to yourself. The most likely result is that the person with the eating problem will feel, *I need to do a better job of hiding what I'm doing, because the people I love are so upset about this.*

What are things I can say that will *provide support?*

When someone we care about is suffering from an eating disorder, we struggle with how to help. We want to charge in, give advice, cheerlead, and fix what is wrong. So often, though, what underlies the eating disorder is something that has made the person you care about feel her life is out of control—some sort of stress or trauma, either from outside in her environment or because of something she is struggling with in her head. The changes in eating behaviors can start as a way to take control or a way to compensate. He may eat a lot to deal with emotions that are difficult to handle. She may feel that the one thing she can control is what she allows into her body—what she eats.

So charging in and taking over—however well-intentioned—can boomerang. They will resist it because, emotionally, they have to. They will rely even more on the compensating strategy they have found—whether it's restricting, bingeing, purging, or exercising. Because once these behaviors develop into an eating disorder, what was a source of control may now also have become something that is controlling. But that is not how they think of it. And even if they do, they will hold even more tightly to it.

How can you approach them, then? Here are some suggestions for parents, grandparents, aunts, uncles, and even older siblings to consider.

- "You've become a really competent, together person. I'm really proud of you. I don't think I'll ever stop being a parent, though, in the sense of having my antennae up and loving you. Those antennae are telling me that something's not okay. I hope you'll talk to me about it when you can."
- "More and more, you are becoming your own person. That's great. Just remember, none of us goes through life alone. And I'll always be there for you."
- "I can feel that something's bothering you, and I know that whatever it is, I can't solve it for you. But maybe I can help make it easier for you to tackle it. I'd like the chance to try."
- "We've always been there for each other before. Please give me a chance to be there for you now."
- "Let's make a pact: to be there for each other when we're all grown-up, the way we've always been while we were kids. No matter how far apart we live or how different our lives are. Okay?"
- "Grown-up problems are a lot tougher to fix. I can't just put a Band-Aid on and say, 'All better!' But I can listen. And maybe

we can brainstorm. Maybe I can help in a different way. I just want you to know that."

- "I might not be the right person to talk to, but maybe I could help you connect with someone who is. Maybe someone who's been in your shoes."
- "I can't help but be worried. That's just who I am. And it's because I think so much of you. Please don't shut me out. Please don't turn me into a fair-weather friend."
- "I love you. It's really hard to see you hurting. It's really hard to sit on my hands and not be able to help."
- "I'm trying to give you space to work this out on your own. Please tell me what else I can do that would help you."

What should I do if my child refuses to eat?

Many children go through periods when they eat very little. A physician can help you determine if your child is basically healthy. But be sure to state plainly that you're concerned. Because physicians often rush through appointments, you may need to say in an assertive way: "I need some time to talk to you about my child. I'm really worried. She isn't eating and she talks about dieting. I'm worried that she is developing an eating disorder. Are you familiar with working with these problems? What can I do?" If your physician is not sure or is unresponsive, you can ask for a referral to someone who knows more about eating disorders. If your doctor is confident that she knows about eating disorders and is clear that your child does not have one, that's great news.

If your child is talking about dieting and is in a normal weight range or is underweight, make clear that dieting is a mistake and that most diets end up resulting in a weight gain. You'll want to help your child see that eating normally and consistently is important for good overall health. If the pattern of dieting continues, talk with a mental health professional who has experience with both children and eating disorders.

What if my child eats too much?

Many children eat when they are bored or when they are lonely, tired, or angry. It usually doesn't help to say, "You eat too much," or "You'll get fat if you keep eating like that." Instead, provide distractions, such as walking the dog, going swimming, painting, writing a poem, learning to knit, building a tree house, making a fort. Keep them busy so their hands have things to do other than eating. You can try saying, "Let's act out a story; who do you want me to be?" or "If you could build something with what we have in this house, what would you like to make?" or "I feel better when I'm moving; shall we dance?" Many kids love karaoke, and it is pretty funny to have someone put on headphones and sing to music others can't hear. In general, offering fun suggestions to children and following the leads you can take from their special interests can lead you not only to lots of fun but also to great ways to avoid passive activities.

Talk about feelings, yours and your child's. Young people usually have trouble finding the "right" words to express what is going on emotionally. Acknowledge just how hard that is, and express your patience and desire to understand. You might say, "I can remember times when it was really hard for me to talk about how I felt, but when I do it sure helps. I'm ready to listen." It sometimes helpful to ask, "Are you feeling angry about that?" or "You seem bored; is that right?" or "Wow, that sure seems like a situation that would make anyone frustrated; how about you?" Learning to voice feelings is often the first step in ending a cycle of stuffing painful feelings down with food.

Most important, model healthy eating. You can point out that we need five to seven servings of vegetables and fruits daily, and encourage your child to have them along with you. If they fill up on the necessary foods, they may be more able to resist unhealthy snacks. Sometimes it helps to say, "You can have what you want after you've had your vegetables and fruits for the day."

Don't keep tempting foods in the house. Teach children to make healthy snacks. There are many kids' cookbooks that have great ideas for after-school or after-dinner snacks. Kids often enjoy the challenge of figuring out how to turn something they don't like into something yummy and healthy.

Children can eat a lot if they also exercise regularly. Families that do active things together help children incorporate exercise into their daily activities.

If your child is overweight and you find it hard to figure out how to engage them in changing their lifestyle to a healthier alternative, consult a professional who can tailor his suggestions to your individual circumstances. Having unique alternatives that match your child's needs is essential to making progress and helping you feel more confident about helping your child achieve healthy eating patterns.

What should I do when my child insists that she must exercise instead of doing other family things?

To an older teenager (or young adult) simply say, "This time is important to me. I respect your commitment to working out, but this activity can't be rescheduled. I expect you to be there." Or, "Sometimes priorities shift, like when I arrange to leave work to come to one of your games, or when Grandma has an important birthday so you have to skip one of your activities." Or, "We do a lot to accommodate the things you need to happen in your life, and we are glad to do that, but sometimes you must find a way to accommodate what we need. You're growing up, and that's a part of it."

If you are the parent of a minor child, you can be more assertive than this. For younger children state your expectations and make clear the consequences of not following the family rules.

Aren't parents supposed to control what their children eat?

Yes and no. Certainly setting reasonable standards is a good idea. But demanding obedience doesn't tend to work. Some young people realize that they hold the power when it comes to deciding what they eat and whether they will keep that food in their system. Power struggles are counterproductive for everyone. If you feel you are in one, you are. Consult a professional who can advise you about how best to extricate yourself from locking horns over food.

What can I say about getting professional help?

Be clear with your child that you want to help her be healthy because you love her and want her to succeed. You can say that you are in over your head and that you would like a professional to help you and her figure out how to evaluate the situation to see if there is a potential for trouble. Point out that:

- Good parents take their kids to an orthodontist when they need braces, even when the child says, "No, I don't want those ugly things on my teeth. And besides, they hurt."
- Parents have an obligation to take their children to professionals when they think they need help.
- You are only doing your job.

Find a professional you trust who can give you support and advice on how to help the young person you are concerned about consider therapy as an option. Please don't try to do this alone; it's too frustrating, lonely, and time-consuming.

Sometimes the direct approach can backfire when talking to kids. They either don't want to admit to having a problem or they don't want to talk about it. So it can help to pave the way. Point out what you are worried about and then ask for clarification. For example, you might try, "It seems to me you are exercising too much. I'm wondering what you think." Or "Tell me more about why you think this is a good idea." In this way you'll find out more about where he is coming from. If you try forcing him out of this, you run the risk of getting into an argument that will only deepen his commitment to maintaining his original position.

What can I say when she says, "I'm fine," or "Don't bother me," or "Leave me alone"?

She is communicating that she is uncomfortable discussing this, or hasn't accepted the need to do so, or is just plain not ready. It could be that she is afraid of what you might say or do. It could be that she fears you will make her feel worse, more ashamed, and guilty. Or that you will take away something she feels she needs to control.

Past experience could be dictating this, too. If talking about this topic has brought pain before, he is not going to be too eager to repeat that experience.

Of course, if they are teenagers, they are also doing what teenagers do, and that is separating from their parents. Because they are trying to hold on to some sort of autonomy by trying to be adult around other adults, they are apt to insist that they know what to do. Even if they don't put these words to their situation, they may see any questions about their behavior as an invasion of privacy or a mark of not being respected as having grown up and able to make their own choices with intelligence.

Still, try explaining what you are worried about. Acknowledge that admitting to an eating problem must feel pretty scary, but that you are open to hearing his opinion and that you hope he might give you a chance to explain your concerns. Try, "I can see this topic upsets you. I can also see that you are suffering, because you are tired all the time and seem so sad. That's not okay. I would like to understand more about how you feel. Can you help me out here?" Or "Maybe this isn't a good time, but can we find another time when it might be better for you? I really want to understand more about what is going on."

What should I say about therapy once she is going?

Once someone is getting professional help there are some appropriate things for family members and friends to say, as well as some inappropriate ones.

When you push someone to talk about what happened in therapy, she won't just feel that this is an invasion of privacy; she may feel guilty for not sharing, or for not letting you help. So it is inappropriate to say:

- "What did you do in therapy today?"
- "What did you talk about?"
- "How did it go?"
- "We just want to know, because we care about you."

Therapy is private and should be respected. If you ask these questions, she will feel pressure to answer and give up that privacy.

Instead, try these kinds of comments. Just don't say these every time he goes:

- "Hope it went okay."
- "If you want to talk, just let me know."

- "If there's anything you want to talk about, I'm here."
- "I'm glad you went."
- "I'm glad you're going to therapy."
- "I'll bet you just want to do something fun right now. Go to it."
- "I don't want to invade your privacy, but I do want to tell you how proud I am that you are working on this. And if you ever want to talk about it, I'll listen."
- "All you've done all day is work. Why don't you kick back for a while before dinner?"
- "I respect that your therapy is private, so I'm not going to ask you about it. But I do want to be there when you need me, so please call on me when you want to."

After a few times, it would be better to say nothing. If you are picking her up from therapy, you could just say, "What do you want to do now?" or "Let's head home."

How about dealing with "grown children"?

Accepting that your control is limited will not only give you more peace of mind, it will also help you have a better relationship with your grown child who is still struggling with an eating disorder. Perhaps the best thing you can do is express your empathy for the problems you observe with comments like:

- "I'm here, and I care."
- "I'm sorry this continues to be hard for you, but I'm willing to listen when you need me."
- "I know I can't fix this for you, even though I wish I could."
- "I'm proud of you for being willing to get help for this problem. I'm with you every step of the way."
- "It means a lot to me that you can tell me how hard this is for you. I'm with you, and I won't try to fix you. Trust me on that."
- "I'm sure you will figure this out over time, and no matter what, I love you!"

Life affords no higher pleasure than that of surmounting difficulties.

∞ —SAMUEL JOHNSON

Chapter Twelve

Managing Emergencies

When we first learn that someone we care about has an eating disorder, it can seem like an emergency. However, this panic often doesn't match the sufferer's sense of the problem. The person with the eating disorder feels like their eating and purging is a way of coping. Eating comfort foods, running for hours, or vomiting after too much to eat are patterns that help manage painful feelings, so the person who has the eating problem is apt to be upset that you think the eating disorder in and of itself is an emergency.

When people react this way it drives most eating problems underground, which leads to more isolation. Unlike emergencies, which require quick action, eating problems tend to be chronic and require repeated interactions over a sustained period, so we have time to measure our responses and think about what comes next.

However, eating disorders do sometimes produce situations that are emergencies and that do require immediate action from those of us who care.

For example:

- Ross passes out during a wrestling match because he didn't eat for three days before the match in order to meet the weight requirements for his classification.
- Leah attempts suicide after her boyfriend tells her he can't deal with her eating disorder.

- Anne perforates her larynx by sticking a fork down her throat because she couldn't seem to make herself vomit by using her finger.
- Rob's heart rate is 220 beats a minute; he is sweating, feels cold, and believes he is going to die. He has been taking a supplement containing the drug ephedra.
- Jana is in danger of financial bankruptcy. All her money goes into purchasing food that she then vomits. She has taken out a loan from a loan shark so that she could hide her behavior and expenses from her husband. She now has severe panic attacks whenever she thinks he'll find out.

What all these situations have in common is that the people's lives could be in danger. That's what makes a situation an emergency.

In this chapter you'll learn the difference between an emergency and a crisis, and you'll learn what do under both circumstances. Here are the most commonly asked questions.

How can I tell the difference between an emergency and a crisis?

An emergency is a situation that requires immediate action because there is a danger to oneself or others.

A crisis is a situation that overwhelms someone's ability to handle their current circumstances. When people aren't coping they panic, they act in highly irrational ways, and they usually appear intensely distressed. Usually what they have done in the past to handle trouble isn't working to resolve the problem at hand. So they don't know what to do to make things better.

Most crises take four to six weeks to resolve to the point that coping is restored and some normal functioning is back in place. During this time the person in crisis often doesn't sleep well or sleeps too much, has trouble eating too much or eats too little, and usually can't focus or concentrate. These patterns make it even harder to cope and resolve problems.

When people are in a crisis their health and safety can be jeopardized. That makes the situation an emergency.

How can I tell whether someone is in crisis?

Most often people in crisis stop functioning in ways that are typical for them. They may appear very distressed, crying or saying things like, "I can't stand this!" or "I feel like I'm going crazy." Or they may say very little and then sleep for long periods without being able to attend to their daily activities. On the other end of the continuum, they might busy themselves with endless activity without doing anything well or appropriately. Usually you will know the person you care about is in crisis because he will behave in ways that are not typical for him.

Is a crisis always a bad thing?

No, often a crisis is just the impetus someone needs to change the destructive things he is doing. In fact, it is not surprising that the Chinese character for crisis includes not only the symbol for distress but also the symbol for opportunity. This is a compassionate way to view crises, because these stressful events are often just what is needed to help the person who is suffering from an eating disorder become more open to getting help.

And your willingness to say that you too are worried and that you believe changes are in order often help the person with the eating disorder see that certain things need to change.

What constitutes a medical emergency?

If the person is unconscious, bleeding, or having trouble breathing, you will need to dial 911 and ask for immediate assistance. Likewise, if the person you care about is threatening suicide or taking some action that could cause harm, you will need to get professional help quickly, and often dialing 911 is the best way to ensure the safety of everyone involved.

If you note any of the following physical symptoms, push for competent medical help to assess the situation:

- seizures (The person may be conscious or unconscious and is either twitching or totally unable to focus. These may last from thirty seconds to several minutes or longer.)

- bradycardia (slow heart rate of less than forty beats per minute)
- irregular heartbeats
- chest pain
- difficulty breathing
- tetany (painful muscle spasms)
- low urine output (less than 400cc per day)
- passing out
- blood in bowel movements
- blood in vomit
- disorientation (not knowing who he is, where he is, or what day it is)
- disordered thinking (not making any reasonable sense)
- talk of suicide

You need to be able to say things such as, "You need to see a doctor soon!" or "I'm really worried, and I can't stand by and do nothing. We are going to the emergency room *now*." In short, any situation that leaves you afraid for someone's overall health should be dealt with by:

- Going to the emergency room of the local hospital
- Calling a suicide-prevention hotline
- Calling the police
- Dialing 911 and asking the operator to connect you to the appropriate referral source.

What if we go to the hospital and I believe the real problem wasn't addressed?

It is quite likely that the underlying problem, the eating disorder, won't be dealt with during the emergency intervention, but that doesn't mean you were wrong to get the person you are worried about emergency help. As long as he is no longer in acute danger, you've done your part to ensure safety.

Later on you can say, "I know you are no longer seeing blood, but we didn't really address your bulimia with the doctor, and I'm worried that if you don't take care of this your health will continue to be in serious jeopardy."

Should we use a medical emergency to force someone into treatment?

Imposing treatment against a person's wishes usually requires extreme measures such as force-feeding by IV, physical or chemical restraints, and restriction of activity. These options are usually very distressing to the people coerced into this kind of treatment. Angry and scared, they will often dig in their heels and do whatever they can to get out of that situation so they can get back to doing things the way they want. Consequently, they often avoid physicians and other health care professionals who they fear will restrict their freedom and choices. Of course, physicians and mental health professionals have to weigh the consequence of forced treatment against death.

Are there legal considerations?

Yes, laws protect adults from being forced to accept treatment they don't want, even when they really need it. Minors and others who are deemed incompetent (a legal term meaning the person is not adult enough or mentally capable of making rational and reasonable choices) may be denied the right to refuse treatment.

If someone is a clear and present danger to herself or others, she can be hospitalized involuntarily against her wishes. But sometimes it seems the only people hospitalized against their will must be screaming that they intend to kill themselves while hanging from an icy ledge. This is because of laws that require treatment to be delivered in the least restrictive manner, and because insurance policies restrict the types of intensive treatment they are willing to reimburse. Nonetheless, police, mental health professionals, and physicians usually know what to do to open the doors for temporary hospitalizations.

Sometimes the only way to help is to get someone who is an adult declared legally incompetent to make decisions. This is a difficult and trying process that often involves going to court. And it should be difficult. This is a last resort. It's much better to get someone to agree to treatment—and the treatment is more likely to help, then, too.

After the emergency is dealt with, what should I say about the eating disorder?

This may be a good time to say that you believe the problems that led to the emergency need to be addressed. Tell her how scared you were for her, how glad you are that she's okay now, and how much you want her to stay that way. Be supportive; be compassionate. Don't use an angry tone of voice. You can best do that by clearly stating what you have observed and then expressing your concern:

- "I'm really scared about what happened last night. I was afraid you were going to be hurt badly. I would feel better if we could talk about how to deal with this more productively. Would you consider professional help?"
- "I'm glad that you regained consciousness and that you are okay now, but I'm worried that your eating problems are causing you to pass out."
- "It scares me to see how you risk your health because of your fears of gaining weight. Don't you think it's time to get help?"

In fact, when someone is in crisis, they are usually more receptive to getting help than when they are just suffering as usual. After they are stabilized, talking about the emergency is usually a good way to talk about "getting better," "doing better," and "feeling better."

IN SUMMARY, WHEN DEALING WITH EMERGENCY SITUATIONS, YOU NEED TO:

- Acknowledge that you need professional assistance
- Find appropriate professionals to help
- Act quickly (call police or 911)
- Get support for you (have someone stay with you or close by to help)

- Do not leave someone alone who is threatening suicide or homicide
- Breathe and remind others to do the same (This may sound silly, but it's the one thing people don't do when they feel panicked and it only makes things worse. A few deep breaths really helps most tense situations.)

Progress, not perfection.

∞—ALCOHOLICS ANONYMOUS SLOGAN

Chapter Thirteen

Handling Lapses—Maintaining Progress

∞

*A*t best, most eating disorders take a long time to get better.

We all wish progress could be quick so the suffering would be less. That once progress is begun that it would continue in a steady, predictable manner. However, this is not the typical course for most eating disorders. Frequently, people move from one eating problem to another as they try something, react to that, and then try something else. For example, someone might move from binge eating to anorexia to bulimia, interspersed with periods where things go pretty well.

Even when we know that these problems take time to change, our hearts ache for consistent progress. But when we, as those most involved with the people who suffer with these problems, get impatient or express our frustration over how long it takes, we only drive people to keep secrets and hide their continued struggles from us. Even when we express our confidence about the future, what the person trying to improve can hear is, "I'm hurting the people I love because I can't get better fast enough."

Each sufferer needs time to:

- see that what he is doing is causing him more trouble than it's solving;
- work out a plan to change those destructive patterns into constructive strategies;

- shift not only eating patterns but also the negative thinking that drives the disorder.

This means we need to find ways to provide support and encouragement over what might be a very long haul. We've given you ideas on how to handle the topics that often come up around eating problems. We hope you'll come to see that one conversation or even multiple conversations won't be enough. Having the patience to provide support during the long process of change, and coping with lapses, is easier when our expectations are optimistic but also realistic.

Here are some answers to the most frequently asked questions about dealing with the long haul of recovery.

How can I express my confidence that things will get better without sounding pushy?

The best way to express confidence in someone who isn't feeling confident is to talk about what you have seen them do in the past to manage and overcome difficult things. Perhaps he quit smoking. Or she went through a divorce. Or he had a child with a drug problem. Or she graduated from college, finished high school, or learned a trade. She learned to swim, manage computer problems, play the piano. Anything you can point out about other accomplishments reconnects the person who is losing confidence to areas where he succeeded.

When you can't think of anything or you don't know the person well enough to come up with examples, you can try questions such as, "Did you ever learn something you initially had a hard time with?" "Were you ever afraid to try something, only to discover it wasn't so bad?" Most people can identify with something they've done that seemed hard but that changed with practice and persistence.

Should I mention that she seems better?

Yes, by all means point out the progress you notice. "You seem happier, and you aren't avoiding family meals. What has this been like for you?" Pointing out what you notice and asking about what seemed to make those accomplishments possible serves two important functions. First, it reaffirms the progress that has been made. And second, it asks them to reflect on what they did to make it better, which strengthens coping skills.

Is it okay to ask if he is better?

Perhaps you haven't noticed much change, but you are concerned about how he is doing. You can say, "We talked about how you were struggling with your weight; how is that going for you?" or "I keep wanting to ask how you are doing with that problem we talked about before. Is it okay to talk about it now?" or "Do you feel like you are getting any better with your eating problems?" If you get some kind of evasive answer or the silent treatment, back off. But many people welcome an invitation to talk about a long-standing struggle, and your question is an expression of your concern and interest in the difficulty of managing an eating disorder. Often, that's appreciated.

Should I ask if she is still getting treatment?

It's okay to ask about treatment if you are prepared to hear the answer without judging. Many people need to take breaks from treatment as they incorporate new ideas or focus on other aspects of life. If your questions reflect respect for her choices and they don't sound judgmental, you will probably be perceived as caring and concerned and she will welcome the opportunity to tell you about why a break was a good idea.

If the person is still in treatment, she may or may not want to talk about what is going on. You can say, "I was wondering how it was going. I haven't asked you about that for a while; is it okay to ask now?" Many people in therapy like to talk about what they are learning and how they are feeling about the process. Others like to mull things over, and find it hard to share unformed ideas with those they care about. Not taking her responses personally will help both of you.

What about the fact that I can't stop worrying that she will start this all over again?

Be patient with yourself. Of course you are worried. Most people even worry that people who are now doing well will "fall off the wagon" and resume the old problems. We especially worry during times of stress or conflict.

It helps to realize that your commitment to the relationship you value is what is most important. And when we accept that whether or not the person we care about has an eating disorder we can still have a good relationship, we don't feel as pressured to "fix it." This acceptance allows us to stay connected without the burden of responsibility for someone else. And that allows us to appreciate the good things we enjoy and focus less on the fears we wish could be relieved.

What can I say when I notice that he seems to be doing the same things that got him into trouble in the first place?

Even when the person you're concerned about realizes that change is necessary and then takes steps to tackle her eating problems, we still feel concern because we know these problems can reemerge.

The term "relapse" is often used to describe the periods when someone who has improved now seems to be struggling with the same old problems. It is often more helpful to think of these periods as lapses rather than relapses. What are some examples of a lapse? It's something like eating too much on vacation, or throwing up one time after having eaten too much, or overexercising during a time of stress.

A "lapse" is a one time event (but it could happen a few times) when most of the time the person is on track with her recovery. "Relapse" is different. That suggests the person you care about is off the track altogether, that it's now back to square one and all progress is lost. This concept is not only depressing; it's also not accurate.

What she learned that allowed her to eat more healthfully is not lost. It's just like remembering how to ride a bike even though years have gone by since the last time you rode. Knowing how to make changes is still there, inside each person who has once made improvements. The knowing isn't gone; it's just dormant. You can remind her of that.

Is she "completely" better if the doctor let her out of the hospital or she was ready to stop day-treatment or some other therapy?

Most people come out of treatment better. Keep in mind that the structure and support that was there during the hospital stay or therapy program are now removed. You can think of this much like the safety net of a trapeze artist. Going without the net is terrifying for most people. They'll have some ideas about how to accomplish their goals but they'll still be full of fear and tension; fear that they'll disappoint those who they hope to impress with their progress, and tension that one false step will lead them right back to where they started. We need to appreciate the strain they're under and remind them of their goals. Remember, "progress not perfection." And that progress can't happen without making tons of mistakes along the way.

Accepting that lapses are part of the recovery process will make things easier for both of you. It will affect your interactions—what you say and do—and it will affect how you both respond. Since she will be under a lot of pressure to make recovery work, you won't want to add to that pressure. She will have a program to follow. Even if you think that program isn't wise or you question some of what she has learned, adopt a-wait-and-see approach.

What if she tells me that her therapist thinks I'm the problem?

Sometimes a person comes out of therapy or the hospital feeling critical of other family members. Sometimes they accuse you of pressures you had no idea you were imposing, other times they describe circumstances you didn't know about. It's hard to feel blamed. That's why we talked about this problem in the first chapter. It helps if you can listen without judging. And that is easier to do when you accept that whatever she is accusing you of is only her perception of what has happened. That doesn't make it reality, but her perception of her circumstances is what matters most to her and her understanding of herself. If you can acknowledge her views, this will deepen your connections and the affection you feel for each other. If necessary, you can reaffirm the importance of being able to maintain affection even if you differ on important perceptions.

This is probably the time to hold your contradictory views in check. You don't want to dilute the core of what she is learning about herself, nor do you want to undermine the insight she is developing and progress she is making.

What if he seems to be giving up? How do I help her recommit to recovery?

No matter how strong they are and how much support you give, there will be times when they will feel like giving up. Or when the eating disorder will feel too safe and comfortable. Like a default position. Remember to use brief encouraging comments. "You'll be okay." "I've seen you do this before." "I know you've done better. What worked in the past?" At these times pose some questions that help them find the hidden reserves they need to keep moving forward.

Consider asking them:

—"Do you want to be 40 (50 or 60) years old and still here?"
—"Do you want to still be doing this ten years from now?"
—"Is this how you see your life?"
—"Don't you want to feel better, you were doing so well?"
—"Didn't you see how much happier you were?"
—"Do you want to spend fifty years regretting what it took five years to do?"
—"What about all the other things you want to do in your life. Don't you want to enjoy all your plans and dreams?"
—"Don't you want to have the strength and endurance to do them?"

What are some things I shouldn't say?

Here are some things that people in recovery reported were said to them that really threw them off—and why.

"You're doing this wrong."

This is not validating. He is trying very hard to climb back to a healthy life and needs all the validation he can get. It's best not to add any new strategies or additional suggestions. Along these lines, don't talk about other people who did something different to get better. Talking about other's successes can set up a feeling of competition or a sense that you expect them to do something they aren't doing.

"We don't think you're continuing to get any better."

You may be trying to say that she needs more help—that the process is stalled or going backward. But it doesn't help to put it in negative terms. Keep in mind that it is normal for progress to be unsteady.

"I can't believe this is happening again."

This is your frustration talking, and it will only make her flinch away. It will feel to her as if you think she is stupid or refusing to listen or not trying hard enough to follow through.

"Are you sure you're really doing okay?"

This sounds so nice and caring, and it is what you feel in your heart, but what he hears is lack of trust in his commitment and no faith in his ability to change. For the same reason it is best not to ask if he is still engaging in such behaviors as throwing up. It's very hard for you, as the friend or family member, to have faith, because you have seen how an eating disorder can make someone manipulative, conniving, and sneaky. But the person working on recovery needs to feel that other people have that faith. That faith will help to sustain his effort.

"I don't understand why you're still seeing a nutritionist. Shouldn't you be done with it by now?"

Actually, professionals do more than provide information and develop a program for someone to follow. Working with a professional over time helps ensure that changes are paced in a manner that is most likely to produce successful results. The person you care about may hear that you think she is not following instructions and that you are concerned that she is wasting time and money by continuing to go.

"You already know everything about the right diet, so shouldn't you be better by now?"

This suggests that knowledge automatically transforms itself into results, that it's just like following a how-to manual or changing the recipes he is going to follow. There's a whole lot more to it than that. Understanding something and being able to do it are two very different things.

"If you don't get it at this point, you never will."

This suggests that one can recover from an eating disorder on his own. Knowledgeable support is vital to the process. It's not a matter of understanding how it works; it's about changing one's thinking so one can change one's actions. He will hear that you don't think he needs any more help and that you are withdrawing support if he can't take this on himself.

"I told you you were losing too much weight!"
Maybe he keeps getting sick or her period becomes erratic, and you want them to take seriously what's happening and recognize they might need to get more help. But no one likes hearing, "I told you so." It doesn't tend to make people receptive to anything else you want to say.

"I thought you were going to start working out and eating well when you got to college."
You may be trying to remind them of what their intentions were and how excited you were about that. But what they hear is that you are disappointed in them and that they are failing everybody.

"If you drop to a size two I'll send you back to the treatment center."
You may be trying to provide an incentive, but this will feel like a threat. Avoid anything that sounds like a threat, because then they won't feel comfortable talking about what is happening, and that means they won't get the support they need or informed intervention if it becomes necessary. Threats will lead to withdrawal and a desire to rebel.

What can I say that might be more helpful?

Most people want to know that you care, that their eating problems haven't alienated you, and that you still have confidence in them and your relationship. Even when you remain worried you can express your support. Here are some words that help.

"Are you stressing out?"
When someone is feeling stress in one area of her life, it is likely to spill over into other areas. So stress can contribute to a lapse, particularly if the eating behaviors are about feeling in control, dealing with emotion, or finding a way to calm down. When you ask about stress, you are not singling out the eating disorder, but rather giving someone the chance to vent, look for solutions, ask for support. If there is stress and behaviors change, don't let it go on too long. If they don't subside in three or

four days, you might want to suggest talking to someone so the pattern doesn't reestablish itself. You could say, "What do you think would help at this point?"

"Do you think you may need to slow down for a while?"

You may have found that the person you care about reads the stress question as code for, "Are you engaging in eating behaviors again?" So this is another way to approach him. Maybe he is juggling a lot of stuff; maybe it's time to assess priorities and see if some things are less important or could be postponed.

"I'm just wondering how everything is going."

This doesn't push for a response. That means she can say "okay" or "fine" or "so-so" and the subject can be dropped. Or she can decide to expand on that and invite a conversation. Either way, you've shown you care.

"I know you are trying to do this on your own, but I'm concerned. Are you okay?"

If you are close, and you have talked about the recovery process, you can express concern. This conveys pride in what he is attempting to do and the suggestion that it is always possible to get support. Yet it ends with a simple question that leaves the decision about any further conversation to the person in recovery. He can cut it short by saying, "Hanging in," or "Thanks for asking," or "It's going okay; what about you?"

"I hate to see you so full of doubt; I wish there were something I could say that would take that away."

Recovery is hard work. Even though someone has been prepared for lapses, they are a lot easier to imagine in theory than to live in real life. They are demoralizing and can make someone doubt herself and her abilities to get through. It helps to acknowledge that. It can make her feelings seem normal and help her find the strength to keep tackling this.

"I hate to see you so down on yourself. It hurts me to watch you do this."

This validates, too. It tells him that you see so much more in him, that you remember when he wasn't that way—that that is more his norm—and that you fully expect him to get back to that place.

"You're so negative about things right now."

If the person you care about has been in therapy that includes behavior modification and other cognitive approaches, this could make him stop and reassess what he is saying or doing and help him switch gears. It's code for saying, "You need to practice what you've been learning about a different way to think."

"What's on your mind? Is something bothering you?"

This is open-ended. And it doesn't ask about recovery or eating or exercise. That can be a relief. It can be tiring if most of one's conversations with most of the people one knows well are about those things. And it can be annoying. People mean well but forget they are not the only ones trying to show support and caring. Talking about other things is refreshing. It says you see a lot more than the eating disorder when you are with her. That you still share the same interests and want to engage in them together, or at least talk about them. That there are other things to focus on and they are all still out there waiting.

"I don't want to lose my child and watch you go through what you went through before. Are you okay?"

This helps a teenager feel she can talk to her parents. It will make her feel that her parents won't get angry and that she can be more open about what is going on and get support.

"Even if you die from this stupid disease, I'm still going to love you. But you'd better not, or I'm going to come and kill you."

This brings humor amidst all the pain. The person who reported hearing this said it made her feel good, and it made her laugh. It helped her to step away from things and get a different perspective.

"Do you want to go do something? Is there something you'd enjoy doing today?" or "Please join us."

It's not uncommon for people with eating disorders to suffer from depression, too. And it's particularly demoralizing to find oneself going backward. This makes it difficult for them to make decisions or to join others in outings and activities. They may keep putting you off and saying no. Don't give up. Don't stop asking. Even it takes a hundred times and months go by. They may want to be there, but know they can't be there emotionally. They may want to join you, but not want to mess up the day for anyone else. Keep trying to include them. Even if they don't go, this will help to make them feel included.

BOOSTERS

When someone is struggling to build self-esteem and confidence, it is a good idea to stop giving specific instructions for what to do and instead express confidence that she already knows what to do and has the skill to do what is necessary. These minimal encouragers are great boosters. When you don't know what else to say, these boosters can help defuse a difficult situation. Most of us have had the experience of being told, "You'll be okay," or "You'll figure that out," and even when we weren't sure, it helped to hear others say they had confidence. Recovery is tough, and it helps to hear how hard we're trying and that our efforts and our successes have been noticed. Here are some positive strokes you can give—both directly to the sufferer and in response to what other people might say about her within hearing distance.

- "I'm so proud of her."
- "I really admire how brave you have been."
- "I'm glad you are working on this. It must take a lot of energy."
- "Be patient. This kind of thing can take a long time."
- "I'm really proud of you for tackling this the way you are."
- "I have so much respect for the way you are tackling this and keeping at it, even though it must be the hardest thing in the world."
- "Don't beat yourself up about this lapse; what you've accomplished so far is amazing and you're going to make it."
- "You have no idea what a trouper he is. I admire his strength and his persistence."

All of us appreciate knowing what we are doing right. We like to know what pleases. So clearly and with caring in your voice, say what you:

- appreciate
- notice that's positive
- have heard others say that is positive
- admire
- notice about the strength it takes to get help
- enjoy about seeing her happier
- aren't worried about
- like about what you see

Compassion brings us to a stop, and for a moment we rise above ourselves.

∞—MASON COOLEY

Chapter Fourteen

Dos and Don'ts—A Helpful Reference

∽

By this time you are probably feeling overwhelmed by all the suggestions of things to say and things not to say about body image, weight, food, exercise, seeking professional help, lapses, blaming and control. This chapter provides an overview and can be used as a quick reference.

Because it can help to see things side by side, every "don't say" is paired with a "do say"—something that will go over better because it is less likely to be taken the wrong way and because it will feel less intrusive, more empathetic, and matter-of-fact.

As long as you say what you would want someone to say to you, as long as you keep in mind how much you respect the person you are talking to, what you say will be supportive and appropriate.

These are only suggestions. These are only a set of guidelines for you to absorb so you can feel comfortable generating your own words.

DON'T SAY	DO SAY
What's wrong with you?!	Something's not right here. Are you okay?
I just don't know what to say to you anymore.	Would it help if I backed off for a while?

DON'T SAY	DO SAY
This is your fault. You need to change.	This isn't about fault. This isn't anyone's fault.
Tell me how to fix this for you.	I'll help you in any way I can.
I can relate. I feel your pain.	I know I can't possibly know what this feels like, what you are going through.
You should be able to control this.	This must all be very hard for you, but I have faith in you.
If you wanted to, you could get back on track.	Part of growing up is making your own choices. I respect that.
You're killing yourself!	I know you've considered all the health implications. I know you are doing the best you can.
How can you do this to yourself?	Maybe this is the best thing for you right now.
I don't care what else is going on; we need to talk right now.	Anytime you want to talk, I'll be happy to sit and listen.
We can't keep avoiding this; we have to talk about this.	Why don't we talk about other things? I'd love to know what's happening in school/at work. What's been happening that's good?
You keep shutting me out.	Sometimes things really get on my nerves. Don't you find that to be true?

DON'T SAY	**DO SAY**
You're wound so tight all the time.	I've been really uptight lately. I need to release some of this tension. Any ideas?
You're being rude to your friends.	Do you feel a need to do this? How come?
I'm the parent.	I can't tell you what to do with your body. That's in your control.
Life is good. Why are you throwing it away?	Life can really stink sometimes, don't you think?
I'm so scared for you.	You're such a strong person. Wherever you want to go, I know you'll get there.
I want to help you.	If you ever want help with something, you can call on me/count on me.
Respect cuts both ways, you know.	I know I don't always show it, but I have enormous respect for you. How you are with other people, how you are with your work. How you take responsibility. How you face up to things. I'll try to do a better job of showing you that. (And I hope you can do that for me, too. I know it's there, but it helps to hear/see it every once in a while.)

DON'T SAY	DO SAY
That dress looks lovely.	That's a really attractive dress.
You look so handsome in that suit.	I really love that fabric.
Wow, you look better.	I bet it's been rough on you.
You're heavier.	It's good to see you.
You're eating so much!	Let's find something good to eat while we talk and catch up on stuff.
You're losing weight. I'm going to send you back to the center.	I don't want to lose my daughter and watch her go through what she went through before. Are you okay?
Is it getting easier?	I understand you've been working really hard.
You look good. Keep doing what you're doing.	I've missed you. What would you like to talk about?
How is it going for you?	I understand you're going through a tough time. Hang in there.
Have you lost weight?	I know you've had a cold. Are you okay?
You look so healthy.	It's great to see you!
Stop cutting me out.	I miss you.
I can't handle hearing about this problem.	This must be hard for you.

Afterword

∞

*T*his book is not a cure-all, but we hope it will continue to help you respond to the various situations that arise—navigate the inevitable ups and downs, find words to fall back on when you come up empty, judge when to push and when to back off, provide the kind of support that can help the people you care about take stock and seek help.

And we hope the book will support you, too. That it will help you: accept that there is only so much we can do—absolve yourself from blame when things aren't going well (and avoid blaming others as well)—gain a deeper understanding of how people's thinking can change when they suffer from an eating disorder—figure out what you can control and what you can't—not lose your life.

We hope this book will help both of you—those of you who struggle to be supportive and those of you who are reaching for recovery.

Additional Resources

PART I

BLAME AND RESPECT

Berry, Carmen Renee & Mark W. Baker. *Who's to Blame?: Escape the victim trap & gain personal power in your relationships.* Colorado Springs, CO: Piñon Press, 1996

Caplan, Paula. *The New Don't Blame Mother: Mending Mother-Daughter Relationships.* New York, New York Routledge. 2000.

Kottler, Jeffery. *Beyond Blame: A New Way of Resolving Conflicts in Relationships.* San Francisco, CA. Jossey-Bass. 1994.

Identity And Self-Respect. Chicago, IL: Great Books Foundation, 1997

MOTIVATION TO CHANGE

Prochaska, James O., Norcross, John C., & DiClemente, Carlo C. *Changing For Good: A Revolutionary Six-Stage Program for Overcoming Bad Habits and Moving Your Life Positively Forward.* New York, New York. Quill. 2002

DiClemente, Carlo C., *Addiction and Change: How Addictions Develop and Addicted People Recover.* New York, New York. Guilford Press 2003

Taking Control of Yourself—Setting Limits

Bower, Sharon A. & Gordon H. Bower. *Asserting Yourself: Updated Edition: A Practical Guide for Positive Change.* Reading, MA. Perseus Books Gp. 1991

Smith, Manuel J. *When I Say No, I Feel Guilty.* New York, New York: Bantom Books, 1975.

Maximizing The Impact of What You Say

Barker, Larry L., Kittie W. Watson. *Listen Up: How to improve relationships, reduce stress, and be more productive by using the power of listening.* New York, New York. St Martin's Press. 2000.

Patterson, Kerry. *Crucial Conversations: Tools For Talking When The Stakes are High.* New York, New York. McGraw Hill. 2002

McKay, Matthew. *Messages: The Communication Skills Book.* Oakland, CA. New Harbinger Pub. 1995.

Merker, Hannah. *Listening: Ways of Hearing in a Silent World.* New York, New York. Harper Collins. 1994.

PART II

Talking About Body Image

Wolf, Naomi. *The Beauty Myth.* New York: William Morrow and Company. 1991.

Johnson, Carol. *Self Esteem Comes in All Sizes: How to Be Happy and Healthy at Your Natural Weight.* Carlsbad, CA. Gurze Books. 2001.

Dixon, Monica. *Love the Body You Were Born With: A 10 Step Workbook for Women.* New York, NY. Berkley Pub Group. 1996.

Cash, Thomas. *Body Image Workbook: An 8 Step Program for Learning To Like Your Looks.* Oakland, CA. New Harbinger. 1997

Erdman, Cheri. *Live Large! Ideas, Affirmations, and Actions for Sane Living in a Larger Body.* San Francisco, CA. Harper Collins. 1997.

Maine, Margo. *Body Wars: Making Peace with Women's Bodies*. Carlsbad, CA. Gurze Books. 2000.

TALKING ABOUT MEDIA

Wallace, Amy. Jamie Lee Curtis: True Thighs. *More* Magazine. September, 2002.

Pope, Harrison G., Katharine A. Phillips, Roberto Olivardia. *The Adonis Complex: The Secret Crisis of Male Body Obsession*. New York, NY. Free Press. 2000.

Grogan, Sarah. *Body Image: Understanding Body Dissatisfaction In Men, Women, And Children*. London; New York: Routledge, 1999.

Doty, William G. *Myths Of Masculinity*. New York: Crossroad, 1993.

TALKING ABOUT TOUCH

Montagu, Ashley. *Touching: The Significance of the Skin*. New York: Harper Row, (1986).

Touch and Feel Puppy. (1999) New York. DK Pub. (a book for pre-schoolers but fun for adults as well)

Zilbergeld, Bernie. (1999) *The New Male Sexuality*. New York. Bantom Books.

Barbach, Lonnie. (1984) *For Each Other: Sharing Sexual Intimacy*. New York. NAL

TALKING ABOUT DIET

Paul Campos. *The Obesity Myth: why America's obsession with weight is hazardous to your health*. New York: Gotham Books, 2004.

LoBue, Andrea & Marsea, Marcus. *The Don't Diet, Live-It! Workbook: Healing Food, Weight and Body Issues*. Carlsbad, CA. Gurze Books, 1999.

Roth, Geneen. *When Food is Love: Exploring the Relationship Between Eating and Intimacy*. New York. Penguin Books, 1991.

Andersen, Arnold, Cohn, Leigh, Holbrook, Thomas. (2000) *Making Weight: Healing Men's Conflicts with Food, Weight, Shape & Appearance.* Carlsbad, CA: Gurze Books, 2000.

TALKING ABOUT EXERCISE

Fitness Fundamentals: Guidelines for Personal Exercise Programs. US Government Document. http://fitness.gov/fitness.html

Schlosberg, Suzanne & Liz Neporent. *Fitness For Dummies.* Foster City, CA: IDG Book, 2000.

Cooper, Kenneth H. *Aerobics Program For Total Well-Being: Exercise, Diet, and Emotional Balance.* New York: E Evans and Company, 1982.

TALKING ABOUT PROFESSIONAL HELP

Yalom, Irvin. *The Gift of Therapy: An Open Letter to a New Generation of Therapists and Their Patients.* New York: Harper Collins, 2002.

WEB PAGES

Center for Mental Health Services
http://www.mentalhealth.samhsa.gov/

National Eating Disorders Association
http://www.nationaleatingdisorders.org/p.asp?WebPage ID=337

Academy for Eating Disorders
http://www.aedweb.org/

National Institute for Mental Health
http://www.nimh.nih.gov/publicat/eatingdisorders.cfm

Books on Eating Disorders
http://www.gurze.com/index.htm
http://eatingdisordersarena.com

No-Diet Information
http://www.dietless.com/
http://www.hugs.com/
http://www.geneenroth.com
http://www.bodypositive.com

Teen Health
http://www.nationaleatingdisorders.org/p.asp?WebPage ID=295

General Health
http://www.mayoclinic.com/
http://familydoctor.org/
http://www.goaskalice.columbia.edu/2357.html

Eating Disorders in Midlife
http://www.mayoclinic.com/invoke.cfm?id=HQ00596

Body Image and Health
http://www.4woman.gov/bodyimage/index.cfm
http://www.about-face.org/
http://www.something-fishy.org
http://www.bodypositive.com

Body Image and Kids
http://www.4woman.gov/bodyimage/kids.cfm
http://www.mirrormirror.com.au
http://www.dadsanddaughters.org/index.html

Body Image and the Media
http://www.mediascope.org/pubs/ibriefs/bia.htm
http://www.about-face.org/

Treatment and Eating Disorders
Many Web sites list treatment options and contain useful information. However, keep in mind that service providers must pay a fee to be listed, so many professionals choose not to advertise in this way. Most sites also claim no responsibility for the credentials and accreditation of those service providers.

For information about psychologists, their credentials and services
http://www.apa.org/

For information about counselors, their credentials and services
http://www.counseling.org
For information about psychiatrists, their credentials and services
http://www.psych.org/
For information about dieticians, their credentials and services
http://www.eatright.org/Public/
For general information from the US government on all professions and
their credentials, try:
http://www.bls.gov/home.htm

Notes and Permissions

∞

<u>NOTES</u>

1. Page xii
Steinem, Gloria. 1992, 1993. *Revolution from Within: A Book of Self Esteem.* Boston: Little, Brown, and Company. P 6

2. Page 5
Heaton, Jeanne, A. 1998. *Building Basic Therapeutic Skills.* San Francisco: Jossey-Bass. P 94.

3. Page 23
Prochaska, J.O. & DiClemente, C.C. (1982) *Transtheoretical Therapy: Toward a More Integrative Model of Change Psycholtherapy.* 20. 161–173. (original source for stages of change)
(more recently)
Prochaska, J.O., Norcross, J.C. & DiClemente, C.C. (1994) *Changing For Good: A Revolutionary Six Stage Program for Overcoming Bad Habits and Moving Your Life Forward.* New York; HarperCollins. P 39.

4. Page 25
Kelly Vitousek "Treatment of Anorexia Nervosa: Enhancing Motivation for Change Across All Stages of Treatment". Workshop Oct 25, 2002 in Columbus Ohio.

5. Page 77
Hellmich, N. (Oct 14, 2003) A Nation Of Obesity. USA Today, McLean, Va. Pg D.07

6. Page 78
Campos, Paul, Jan 13, 2003. *Why being fat isn't bad for you. Weighting Game.* New Republic. P 17–21.

7. Page 78
Periello, V.A. (September 2001) "Aiming For A Healthy Weight In Wrestlers And Other Athletes." Contemporary Pediatrics. 2001; 9:55 Published by Medical Economics Company at Montvale, NJ 07645-1742

8. Page 96
www.NationalEatingDisorders.org
"Statistics: Eating Disorders and their precursors."
http://www.nationaleatingdisorders.org./p.asp?WebPage_ID=286&Profile_ID=41138
"Some Facts About the Media's Influence in Our Lives."
http://www.nationaleatingdisorders.org/p.asp?WebPage_ID=320&Profile_ID=41166

9. Page 98
Amy Wallace. (September, 2002). "True Thighs." *More Magazine*, p 90–95.

10. Page 118
Satter, Ellyn. (1987) *How To Get Your Kid to Eat . . . But Not Too Much,* Palo Alto, CA Bull Publishing. p60 & p69.

11. Page 121
"The Big Deal About Dieting: What You Should Know"
http://www.nationaleatingdisorders.org/p.asp?WebPage_ID=320&Profile_ID=41162

12. Page 121
Bennet, W. & Gurin, J. (1982) *The Dieter's Dilemma: Eating Less and Weighing More.* New York, Basic Books.

13. Page 122
Lissner, L., Odell, PM, D'Agostino, RB, Stokes, J., Kreger, BE, Belanger, AJ, Brownell, KD (June 1991) Variability of body weight and health outcomes in the Framingham population. New England Journal of Medicine. Vol 324: 1839–1844.

14. Page 127
Samara J. & Popkin, B. (Jan 22/29, 2003) Patterns and Trends in Food Portion Sizes, 1977–1998. Journal of the American Medical Association. Vol 289, #4. p450–453.

15. Page 127
Partial list of "Dangerous Supplements" Consumer Reports May 2004 issue of. © 2004 by Consumers Union of U.S., Inc. Yonkers, NY 10703–1057. p15.
http://www.consumerreports.org/main/content/display_report.jsp?FOLDER%3C%3Efolder_id=419341&ASSORTMENT%3C%3East_id=333141&bmUID=1112236276632

16. Page 131
Adler, J & Underwood A. "Health for Life, Starve Your Way to Health" Newsweek, Jan 19, 2004. p 46

17. Page 145
"Benefits of Regular Exercise." From Exercise: A Healthy Habit to Start and Keep." [n/a-author(s); http://familydoctor.ort/x2801.eml: October 2003.]

18. Page 145
Fitness Fundamentals: http://fitness.gov/fitness.html p 2

19. Page 163
http://www.something-fishy.org/dangers/dangers.php
Section entitled "Physical dangers of eating disorders" Copyrighted by

Something Fishy [Music & Publishing] Amy Medina, <u>Fishmaster@ something-fishy.com</u>. All rights reserved. Reprinted with permission.

PERMISSIONS

We want to thank the following for granting permission to include their copyrighted material:

Page 96
"Statistics: Eating Disorders and their precursors." "Some Facts About the Media's Influence in Our Lives."
Copyright by and reprinted with permission from: National Eating Disorders Association.
(<u>www.NationalEatingDisorders.org.</u>)
"Statistics: Eating Disorders and their precursors."
http://www.nationaleatingdisorders.org/p.asp?WebPage_ID=286& Profile_ID=41138
"Some Facts About the Media's Influence in Our Lives."
http://www.nationaleatingdisorders.org/p.asp?WebPage_ID=320& Profile_ID=41166

Page 118
"What is Normal Eating?"
Copyright by and reprinted with permission from Ellyn Satter's *How to Get Your Kid to Eat...But Not Too Much,* 1987. Bull Publishing, Palo Alto, CA 1987. For ordering information, call 800-676-2855 or see <u>www.ellensatter.com</u>

Page 127
Partial list of Dangerous Supplements as published in the May 2004 issue of Consumer Reports. © 2004 by Consumers Union of U.S., Inc. Yonkers, NY 10703-1057, a nonprofit organization. Excerpted with permission from the May 2004 issue of Consumer Reports® for educational purposes only. No commercial use or reproduction permitted. <u>www.ConsumerReportsOnHealth.org</u>, <u>www.ConsumerReports.org</u>.

Page 131
From "Starve Your Way to Health", By Jerry Adler and Anne Under-
wood. 1/19/2004. From Newsweek, 1/19/2004 ©[2004] Newsweek Inc.
All rights reserved. Reprinted with permission.

Page 145
Section entitled "Benefits of Regular Exercise" from "Exercise: A
Healthy Habit to Start and Keep" [n/a-author(s); http://familydoctor.
org/x2801.xml; October 2003].

Page 163
Section entitled "Physical dangers of eating disorders" Copyrighted by
Something Fishy [Music & Publishing] Amy Medina, Fishmaster@
something-fishy.com. All rights reserved. Reprinted with permission.
http://www.something-fishy.org/dangers/dangers.php